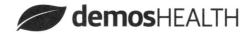
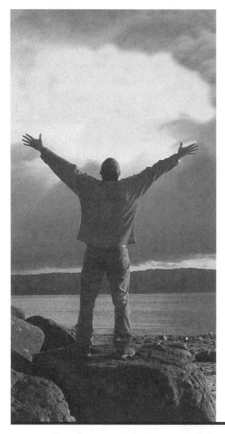

Stronger After Stroke

Your Roadmap To Recovery

PETER G. LEVINE

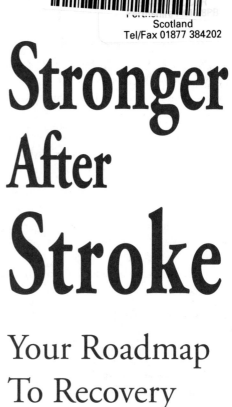

demosHEALTH

Visit our web site at www.demosmedpub.com

Medical information provided by Demos Health, in the absence of a visit with a health-care professional, must be considered as an educational service only. This book is not designed to replace a physician's independent judgment about the appropriateness or risks of a procedure or therapy for a given patient. Our purpose is to provide you with information that will help you make your own health-care decisions.

The information and opinions provided here are believed to be accurate and sound, based on the best judgment available to the authors, editors, and publisher, but readers who fail to consult appropriate health authorities assume the risk of any injuries. The publisher is not responsible for errors or omissions. The editors and publisher welcome any reader to report to the publisher any discrepancies or inaccuracies noticed.

Special discounts on bulk quantities of Demos Medical Publishing books are available to corporations, professional associations, pharmaceutical companies, health-care organizations, and other qualifying groups. For details, please contact:

Special Sales Department
Demos Medical Publishing
386 Park Avenue South, Suite 301
New York, NY 10016
Phone: 800-532-8663 or 212-683-0072
Fax: 212-941-7842
E-mail: rsantana@demosmedpub.com

Library of Congress Cataloging-in-Publication Data
Levine, Peter G.
   Stronger after stroke : your roadmap to recovery / Peter G. Levine.
      p. cm.
   Includes index.
   ISBN-13: 978-1-932603-74-3 (pbk. : alk. paper)
   ISBN-10: 1-932603-74-3 (pbk. : alk. paper)
   1. Cerebrovascular disease. 2. Cerebrovascular disease—Patients—Rehabilitation. 3. Self-care, Health. I. Title.
   RC388.5.L48 2009
   616.8'1–dc22

                                                                                          2008026248

Made in the United States of America

10   11   5   4

CONTENTS

Safeguarding the Recovery Investment 47

Cool Treatment Options 67

Elements of Exercise Essential to Recovery 99

Recovery Strategies 113

PREFACE

Every stroke survivor has a certain level of potential recovery. Few reach that potential. Stroke survivors who reach their potential do so because they have *no choice*. This breed of "super-survivor" is so unwilling to let go of their career, their independence, or a personal passion that they are compelled to recover. They intertwine recovery with what they love to do. Sometimes recovery is so much a part of what they love doing that they don't even notice they're recovering!

For the super-survivor, recovery is a vision quest. The challenge of recovery is no different from other challenges they've conquered in life. They get on with it. They put in the time. They fall in love with the process. In much the same way athletes and musicians enjoy practice, stroke survivors who recover see the process of recovery as an opportunity for growth.

This book is designed to meld the spirit of these unusual survivors with the latest and greatest recovery research. In this book you will find a list of suggestions that will jump start the process of *embracing recovery*.

In the mid-1800s, scientists began mapping the brain. Each portion of the brain was segmented. Each section was declared as the *only* possible site for everything from the ability to do math to moving your toes. Researchers asserted that one section, on the left side of the brain, controlled speech, another section at the top of the brain, movement. The back of the brain processed vision, the front solved problems. Mapping suggested that the brain was static and forever fixed, frozen, and locked. This was stark news for stroke survivors. What happened, for instance, if the stroke killed the language portion of the brain? Because science thought the brain unchangeable, attempting to use different parts of the brain for language was *un-*

thinkable. Once language or limb movement, or sensation, or anything else was damaged by the stroke, it was gone, forever.

There is good news however: These scientists were wrong!

Recent research has revealed a remarkable attribute of the brain—flexibility. The brain can be rewired and, under certain conditions, radically rearranged. One hundred billion neurons strong, the brain can be changed into whatever kind of tool we want. And there is more good news: The process of rewiring the brain is incredibly simple.

Although the brain is the most complex entity in the known universe, it responds and changes according to simple instructions. All a person needs to do to change his or her brain is a whole lot of focused and dedicated practice. And it happens fast. Large portions of our brains can be rewired in a matter of hours, days, or weeks. Understand: This is not some sort of vague concept; this is an actual physical event, measurable by brain-scanning technology. The brain, in short, can be worked just like muscle. From learning to control emotions to hitting a baseball, the core of change involves rewiring the brain. You might suspect that there is a bit more to it, and there is. While the idea of "practice makes perfect" is simple, *how* to practice is more complicated. This book defines the time needed to drive neuroplastic change. Rewiring the brain also involves another rather large pink elephant in the room: Motivation. Neuroplasticity (the scientific word for brain rewiring) takes a tremendous amount of work. It does not necessarily involve a long period of time, just a lot of effort.

Your hard work is the most essential aspect of successful recovery. Clearly, *the most important person involved in the recovery from stroke is you.* Much of the work can be done at home with help from family and friends while under the guidance of doctors and therapists. And while clinicians are essential to the recovery process, you and your caregivers should not wait for health professionals to chaperon you toward your highest level of potential recovery. There is no doctor, therapist, minister, guru, or shaman in a better position to run your master recovery plan. There is no one who cares as much. Accept the challenge, empower yourself, focus on recovery, work hard, don't give up, and watch an upward spiral emerge that allows for the highest level of recovery.

I wrote this book because I couldn't figure out why it hadn't already been written. So much has been revealed by research in the last decade or so, and stroke survivors weren't receiving the information. If you searched magazines and the Internet you might obtain a smattering of related information. But there was no singular source. *Stronger After Stroke* is a "field manual" of information unifying and simplifying most of what is currently known about recovery. The word *most* is emphasized here because one of the clear messages of this book is held within the proverb: "You can give a man a fish and feed him for a day. Or you can teach a man to fish and feed him for a lifetime." Recovery requires knowing the latest and greatest research. Appendix I includes quick and easy ways of discovering what is new and effective in stroke-recovery research. Billions have been spent on stroke-recovery research. You should benefit.

INTRODUCTION

We are what we repeatedly do.
—Aristotle

In the last decade or so, stroke-recovery research has focused on a few basic core concepts. Understanding these building blocks of recovery will help you decide which of the growing number of treatment options is right for you. All of the following will give you insight into your recovery planning.

Elements Essential to Recovery From Stroke

Mixing the following elements has been shown to the drive neuroplastic (brain rewiring) change necessary for recovery:

1. **Repetitive**. Pick options that use **repetitive practice**. Movements that you want to relearn have to be performed over and over. For instance, if you want to lift your foot better, then you would concentrate on doing that movement repeatedly and with the highest possible quality of movement. Use of repetition requires "nipping at the edges" of your current ability. With each attempt, try to extend beyond your present ability a little bit more.

2. **Task specific. Neuroplastic** (brain rewiring) change is much more likely to occur if the movement that you are trying to relearn is part of a real-world task. The task has to be meaningful (important, essential, engaging) to you. The more important the task is to you, the more it will drive recovery. For instance, if you are

trying to regain the ability to pick up objects, make it part of a real-world task that is meaningful to you. If you love to paint, practice picking up a paintbrush. But what if you can't pick up a paintbrush? You only need to practice a portion of the task. It is not necessary to have the ability to accomplish the entire task to make it task specific. If the task is picking up a cup, you may only be able to get the hand to the table but not be able to actually grasp the cup. As you bring the hand up to the table, have a cup there to provide an obvious goal.

3. **Massed practice**. In rehabilitation clinics, therapy is usually scheduled as distributed practice. This sort of schedule involves relatively short sessions (15 minutes to 2 hours) distributed over a long period of time (weeks, months, years). Massed practice schedules involve sessions that last 5 to 8 hours, but the sessions are distributed over a short period of 1 to a few weeks. Research indicates that massed practice produces much more of the vital sort of brain rewiring needed to recover from stroke.

4. **Novel**. Work on movements that are novel (new) to you. Of course, the movements are not really *new*. You may have been doing the movements for 50 years prior to your stroke. But it is considered novel if it has yet to be learned since your stroke. Researchers use the word "novel" but a better word may be "challenging." Focus on re-learning challenging movements. Attempting movements that are too easy will not help you recover. As soon as you can perform a movement at a quality that reaches about 80% of your prestroke ability, move on to another novel movement.

The P.E.N.S. Concept

The P.E.N.S. concept provides an effective way to decide whether or not an option is worthy of consideration. It includes:

P is for *Patient driven*. Can you do the therapy by yourself, or does it require supervision? Does it require a lot of training, or is it difficult to understand? You should find out if the recovery option has the potential to be used at home, relatively easily, and with little cost and set-up.

E is for ***Evidenced based***. Has the option been researched? Some therapies have never been tested. Some that have been tested have not done well. Some therapies have been tested in small, poorly run studies. When researching the recovery option, ask the question: Did it shine or was it a lemon?

N is for ***Neuroplastic***. Does the recovery option promote neuroplastic change? That is, will it rewire the brain in a way that helps recovery? The problem is, science may not have yet proven that the option you've chosen actually rewires the brain. There are few recovery options that have been tested this way. Try to determine if the therapy has all the earmarks of neuroplasticity included in Essential Elements of Recovery From Stroke discussed in the previous section.

S is for ***Simulations vectors***. This is a fancy way of saying, "Consider all options as you plan your recovery." There is no one magic bullet for stroke recovery. Therapists tend to use a small group of therapies that they know well. Researchers tend to focus on a small group of related treatment options. Both therapists and researchers bring important perspectives to stroke recovery. But in some ways, both lack a sufficiently broad perspective. When stroke recovery is viewed globally, a hidden secret emerges: *It's not anything, it's everything.* Imagine stroke recovery as a picture puzzle. Solving the stroke-recovery puzzle involves using the puzzle pieces (recovery options) to build as complete a picture as possible. If the puzzle is done correctly, the highest possible level of recovery is achieved. The stroke-recovery puzzle has two added dimensions that other picture puzzles don't:

    1) The number of pieces (treatment options) is continually expanding.

    2) The background picture (where you are in the recovery arc) changes.

Finding out what piece fits where and when these pieces fit is the most important part of your recovery plan.

Good News and Bad News

Recovery takes hard work and commitment. It's not easy. Simply, it will most likely be the hardest thing you've ever done.

- *The good news*: The process of recovering from stroke is both intuitive and simple.
- *The bad news*: Recovery takes a lot of hard work.

If someone is telling you that they can help you recovery and they have special ways of doing it without you working hard, grab your wallet and leave!

While limbs on one side of the body are most impacted, research has found that all four limbs are affected by the brain damage caused by stroke. Because all four limbs are affected, researches use the terms "more affected" and "less affected" when describing the relative deficit in the limbs after stroke. Please note that for the sake of brevity and simplicity, this book sometimes uses the following terms:

- "Bad" — the limbs more affected by the stroke.
- "Good" — the limbs less affected by the stroke.

These terms are not meant to reflect the potential for recovery, nor the relative importance of the limb.

ACKNOWLEDGMENTS

I would like to thank the following:

My wife, Aila, for the many, many conversations we had about stroke recovery and for all of her support during the 3 years it took to write this book.

Dr. Stephen J. Page, my friend and boss, for encouraging colleagues and stroke survivors alike with a belief that we can change things and should be unafraid in doing so; the members of the Kessler Medical Rehabilitation Research and Education Corporation's Human Performance Movement Analysis Lab (1999-2003) for teaching me the nuts and bolts of clinical research; the members of our lab, the Neuromotor Recovery and Rehabilitation Laboratory, located at the Drake Center and under the auspices of the University of Cincinnati; my mom, Rosemarye Levine for helping me to read before I went to school and helping me to write once I got there; my dad, Martin Levine, for asking me the best question a confused writer can be asked: "What are you trying to say here?"

I would also like to acknowledge all the stroke survivors I've talked to over the past decade, each with their unique story and their individual contribution.

Stronger After Stroke

Stroke Recovery Essentials

PLAN YOUR WORK AND WORK YOUR PLAN

Every great journey starts with a great plan. An ambitious recovery plan is vital to your recovery. The plan begins to evolve in the hospital, right after the stroke, and it continues to develop during your time involved in:

- skilled nursing facilities
- rehabilitation hospitals
- outpatient clinics
- home therapy

This early portion of the plan is easy because therapists are developing and implementing the plan. What do you do after occupational, physical, and speech therapies are ended? Stroke survivors typically face the rest of their lives, and the rest of the struggle toward recovery, with no formal recovery plan. Once the standard therapies have ended, the power of your plan becomes even more vital. This is a critical time in recovery. There are three options you can choose from:

1. You believe that, because your therapy has ended, your recovery has ended.
2. You are willing to continue your recovery, but you are not sure what to work on. You decide that you'll join a gym and see what happens.
3. You develop a plan that takes you to the highest level of recovery possible. You know that your plan will change over time. Your plan has built-in goals. Achieving goals gives rise to new goals and new achievements. This forces an upward spiral of recovery.

HOW IS IT DONE?

A powerful and successful recovery plan will:

- *Be measurable*: The recovery plan includes specific goals and landmarks that represent breakthroughs in the recovery process. These breakthroughs are predicted by the plan. The same way coaches set goals for athletes, your plan should set goals that promote recovery. Examples of measurable goals include:
  — "I will be able to walk 50 yards at my daughter's wedding in 3 months."

— "I will be able to use a fork and knife by Christmas."
— "I will be able to pull rope, hand over hand, on my sailboat by next summer."

- *Be flexible*: Stroke recovery involves a constantly shifting set of opportunities. The choice of recovery options and exercises that you'll use will change as you recover. A flexible recovery plan allows for quick adjustments to promote further recovery. For instance, consider the goal, *"I will be able to pick up a cup with my bad hand."* Once you are able to do this, the plan is adjusted to provide a new challenge (e.g., *"I will be able to pick up and drink from a cup"*). The goal is made more difficult to promote even more recovery.
- *Encourage self-reliance*: Focus on recovery techniques that you understand and can carry out yourself. When you can perform the recovery technique without the aid of a clinician, you enter a whole new level of recovery. Promoting self-reliance allows you to recover even after formal therapies have ended. This Do-It-Yourself spin on recovery allows you to take control of the process.
- *Include short- and long-term goals*: A short-term goal is to walk 10 feet. A long-term goal is to walk without a limp. The long-term goal is made with the series of short-term goals in mind. As a metaphor, the short-term goals are bricks. The long-term goals are the blueprints for a brick house.

WHAT PRECAUTIONS SHOULD BE TAKEN?

Any plan should be done within parameters of safety. Consider the examples, "I will be able to walk a quarter mile in 10 minutes, and I will accomplish this by Christmas." Walking long distances has obvious inherent risks. On the other hand, a goal like, "I will be able to open my hand enough to grasp a cup handle within the next month" may rely simply on repetitions of opening and closing the hand, and so contains little risk. The task involved and the skill level needed will determine the level of precaution. "Safety First" is essential to the recovery process because nothing stops recovery like an injury.

✳   ✳   ✳

SAY NO TO PLATEAU

Therapists will stop treating you when they can no longer measure improvement. This lack of progress toward recovery is commonly called a **plateau**. Plateau means "flattening out." From the stoke survivors point of view, the act of ending treatment says "That's it. You won't get any better." In many stroke survivors this has an unfortunate dual effect. First, the end of therapy means the end of the support, guidance, and expertise of therapists. Second, saying that a stroke survivor is no longer making progress often (but thankfully not always) becomes a self-fulfilling prophecy. The stroke survivor thinks, "The professionals who know the most about stroke recovery believe that I'm not going to make any more progress. I guess that's all I can expect." This assumption is not correct. There are several reasons for mistaken assumptions about when recovery has ended.

- Health-care professionals have sometimes purported that during the **chronic** stage of stroke (after the first 3 months to 1 year) no further recovery can be made. The truth is that stroke survivors can continue to make progress years, even decades after their stroke.
- To save money, payers (insurance, Medicare, etc.) put pressure on therapists to end therapy as soon as possible. Therapists would prefer to treat stroke survivors for longer periods, but they cannot. The result is that therapy is usually ended before the fullest possible recovery is realized.
- The tests that therapists use are often not sensitive enough to detect small but important changes in recovery. For instance, tests of spasticity and reflexes can indicate progress toward recovery, but these two tests are rarely done in therapy settings. Also, payers accept data from a small group of tests. The question is: Is there really no progress, or are the wrong tests being used?
- New therapy techniques, no matter how effective, are not used for one of the following reasons:
  — Lack of therapist training in the new therapy
  — Lack of support for the therapy by the rehabilitation facility
  — Payers do not pay for the therapy
  — Clinicians are unaware of the therapy
  — The therapy does not make a profit

- Simply, your recovery could progress, but the most effective therapy is not available in the typical therapy settings.
- Survivors and their families often push for release from the rehab facilities as soon as possible. Therapists are sensitive to this. Therapists work to help patients get as safe and as functional as quickly as possible. Rushing the survivor through the system means:
  — Less time is spent recovering
  — Less guidance is available
  — Less recovery is attained
- Therapists focus on helping you become functional and safe. **Functional** is defined as the ability to do useful or practical activities. For instance, if you can dress yourself, even if you don't use you "bad" arm and hand, you are considered functional in dressing. Walking safely, even if it involves a cane and orthosis on your foot, is considered functional walking. Being functional will get you home and help you get on with your life. But being functional does not usually represent the highest possible level of recovery you can achieve. Achieving the highest possible level of recovery requires extending beyond functional ability.

The word **plateau** has been used by clinicians to describe the point at which "no further recovery can be made." But not everyone considers a plateau a negative thing. Athletes have used the word for decades. A plateau to an athlete is different from the way plateau is used to describe the end of recovery after stroke. Athletes consider a plateau as a point in their training where their present training techniques no longer help them get better, stronger, or faster. Athletes respond to a plateau by trying new strategies to improve their ability. Stroke survivors should view a plateau the same way athletes do; as an opportunity to reevaluate, rejuvenate, and recalibrate.

HOW IS IT DONE?

Many of the suggestions in this book can help you overcome temporary plateaus. A general rule is to assume that there will be no lasting plateau. Assuming no limits to recovery may be optimistic but it allows for the largest opportunity for the highest level of recovery. If you want to get better, assume you will return to the same level of ability you enjoyed prior to the stroke. You may not achieve full recovery, but you'll still have extended farther than the supposed plateau.

If your recovery efforts are not producing results, a temporary plateau will follow. When this happens, and it will, do what athletes do, and change your training techniques. Challenge your **physiatrist** and therapists with suggestions of techniques, treatments, and technologies that you find during your research. If you see something that you think might work, ask these clinicians to use them. Remember: therapy was most likely stopped because these health professionals believed that recovery ended. If therapists just continued to use the same techniques then, indeed, you would not improve further. The same techniques will likely generate the same results. In your own attempts toward recovery look for new recovery options that might work.

WHAT PRECAUTIONS SHOULD BE TAKEN?

There are some instances where stroke survivors cannot achieve any more movement than they have at a given point in time. This is usually the case only when the stroke survivor does not have the mental capacity to try.

✳   ✳   ✳

USE YOUR FANTASTIC PLASTIC BRAIN

Here are some "mind blowers":
- The human brain is the most complex structure in the universe.
- There are 100 billion neurons (nerve cells) in the brain.
- A typical stroke kills less than 2 billion neurons.

But those numbers are small compared to the number of connections between neurons in the brain. There are an astounding quadrillion (a thousand trillion) connections between neurons. This is good news for stroke survivors. The number of connections between neurons is more important than the number of neurons. Forging new connections between the neurons that survive is the basis for all recovery from stroke.

Recovery will naturally follow from working with the one organ damaged by the stroke and from which all true recovery comes: the brain. In order to recover, stroke survivors have to rewire their brain. The technical term is **neuroplasticity**. All true recovery from stroke involves rearranging the neurons (nerve cells) of the brain.

Neuroplasticity is a long word that, like so many medical words, can be broken down to determine the meaning. "Neuro" basically means having to do with nerves. The second half of the word is *plasticity* (from the, Latin, *plasticus* which means *molding*). The root word is plastic. Plastic, when it is heated, becomes flexible and can be molded into almost any shape. Together *neuro* and *plastic* comprise the word neuroplastic.

This concept, that the brain is moldable according to the will and actions of the individual, is not on the cutting edge of stroke recovery therapy, *it is the cutting edge*. Neuroplastic change happens in all of us, all the time, and happens without us knowing a neuron from a necktie.

One of the proven ways to rewire the brain is called **repetitive practice**. Repetitive practice involves repeatedly practicing a movement, even if you can only do a small part of that movement. One of the things that stroke survivors often ask is, "How many times do I have to attempt a movement before I see improvement?" Or, "How many repetitions do I have to do before I rewire my brain?" There is no specific number that will always answer this question. Some scientists have tried to guess the number. 10,000 repetitions is the number often suggested. Others have proposed 140,000 as the number. The number is also not known for someone who has not had a stroke. To become a high-level expert at something (i.e., a professional basketball player, carpet weaver, or musician) the numbers of repetitions needed are between 1 and 2 million. But computing the number for stroke survivors is tricky. The number would vary from one stroke survivor to the next depending on:

- The complexity of the movement to be relearned
- The amount of movement currently available
- The intensity and focus with which the repetitions are done

HOW IS IT DONE?

You are the only person who can rewire your brain. The best therapist in the world can't accomplish this for you. Neuroplasticity, and the recovery that results, emerges from the inside out. The more movement initiated, the more repetitions of a movement attempted, the more voluntary effort made, the more the brain has a chance to rewire, reconfigure, and rebuild.

Neuroplasticity happens fast. There are classic experiments in neuroscience (the science that deals with nerves) that prove that large portions of the brain can be rewired with little more than 4 days of dedicated work. There is a catch, however. Rewiring the brain after stroke requires hard and focused work. Some stroke survivors may not have the cognitive ability or the mental focus required to rewire their brain using neuroplasticity. This is usually because the stroke survivor has lost the ability to *try*. In short, when the stroke survivor *tries*, over and over, that effort rewires the brain.

Neuroplastic change happens to all of us, all the time. The smallest event, from humming a tune to catching a set of keys, will cause neuroplastic change. But if a skill is developed with the right intensity, it will promote lasting change in the brain that will drive the recovery process. The saying among scientists who examine how the brain works is "neurons that fire together wire together." Here is how this concept works. Imagine you are standing on the beach, 10 feet from the water's edge. You have a bucket of water, and you pour the water toward the ocean. You pour the first bucket of water. It flows a few inches and then becomes absorbed by the sand. The second bucket travels a foot or two. The third bucket extends even further. After a few more buckets of water, you have formed a creek to the ocean. All the water that you pour from then on flows easily to the sea. Neurons (nerve cells) in the brain work much the same way. Every time you move, you forge new connections to make that movement easier and easier until you can perform the movement without thinking.

Neuroplastic change is the result of the same set of neurons in the brain firing, over and over, in the same way. The process needed to rewire your brain docs not need to be fully understood to benefit from its power. Simply, the brain can be treated like a "black box." If you put in the right kind of focused, repetitive effort, you get out better movement. The tools used to communicate with the brain during recovery from stroke are the affected limbs. That is, actively moving the limbs will rewire the brain. The increased coordination in the limbs will be the proof positive that your brain is being rewired. This is why accurately measuring progress by testing the amount and quality of limb movement is so important. If there is neuroplastic change, that change will be reflected by better movement.

Neuroplasticity is something that musicians and athletes know well because they know the value of focused practice. The same efforts that help athletes and musicians become the best they can be can help stroke survivors rewire their brains to navigate around the area of brain tissue killed by the stroke. If enough of this rewiring occurs, the stroke survivor can make progress even when she is in the chronic stage (more than 6 months to a year after stroke) of recovery. Research, with the aid of magnetic resonance imaging (MRI) has proven that the brain can essentially rewire. Other sophisticated tests (kinematics, kinetics, **electromyography**, and other outcome measures) have shown a direct link between this rewiring and improvements in the ability to move and function.

The trick to rewiring the brain after stroke is finding the sort of therapies that promote neuroplastic change. The tools that are helpful in changing your brain neuroplastically range from highly sophisticated robots (see Recovery Machines, page 169) to simple **repetitive practice**. Other strategies outlined in this book including **bilateral training** (see The Good Trains the Bad—Bilateral Training, page 93), **constraint-induced therapy** (CIT), (see Constraint-Induced Therapy for the Arm and Hand, page 68), and **mental practice** (see Imagine It!, page 78) will drive rewiring of the brain.

WHAT PRECAUTIONS SHOULD BE TAKEN?

The level of commitment needed to rewire your brain requires the guidance of your doctor. Safety is essential. Many of the concepts in this book ask for an increased amount of time dedicated to recovery. Increased time requires increased muscle, heart, and lung effort. Brain rewiring also requires sustained focus and a level of emotional commitment that can be stressful physically and mentally. Focused effort toward neuroplastic change requires an elevated focus on safety. Neuroplasticity is fatiguing because it is a physical process, much like building and reshaping muscles. But rewiring the brain also involves muscles working in ways to which they are not accustomed. So rewiring the brain involves fatigue from both building your muscles and changing your brain. Fatigue can lead to unsafe efforts and unsafe decision-making. Be careful as you change your fantastic plastic brain.

✳   ✳   ✳

A DOCTOR MADE FOR STROKE SURVIVORS

There are many types of doctors that can help folks that have had stroke—from neurologists to primary care physicians. But there is one kind of medical doctor who has specific training in stroke recovery: **physiatrists** (fizz EYE uh trists). Their medical training and special knowledge of stroke recovery make physiatrists vital to the process of recovery.

Physiatrists are often called "stroke doctors" because they are the medical professionals that patients most often associate with treatment for impairments caused by stroke. Physiatrists:

- Know the latest stroke-related medical treatments and will be able to prescribe the most appropriate medications
- Do special testing that will help determine where you are in your recovery
- Are able to design a recovery plan that focuses on the medical side of recovery, including spasticity reduction and pain control
- Have a large number of tools at their disposal to help foster the continuation of recovery from stroke

HOW IS IT DONE?

After their therapy ends most stroke survivors never visit a physiatrist again. In fact, most stroke survivors don't even remember what a physiatrist is, a few years past their stroke. Because of this lost relationship, survivors are unaware of years of medical advancements that can impact their recovery. I even have a joke about it: *When a stroke survivor is asked, a couple of years after his stroke who his physiatrist is, he responds, "There's nothing wrong with my feet!"*

Ask your primary care physician for a referral to a physiatrist. Get recommendations from other stroke survivors. Look for an aggressive physiatrist who is willing to work with you as you actively strive toward full recovery. Visiting a physiatrist can help set up an upward spiral in your recovery. For instance:

- You visit a physiatrist.
- The physiatrist treats your spasticity.
- Since your spasticity has reduced, the physiatrist writes a prescrip-

tion for therapy to help build on movements unmasked by your newly loosened muscles.
- The reduction in spasticity combined with therapy leads to recovery of lost movement.
- Recovery of lost movement allows you to challenge yourself with other new movements.

A visit to a physiatrist will often trigger a prescription for more therapy. There are several other reasons to see a physiatrist that may or may not be directly related to recovery from stroke. The following should automatically trigger a visit to a physiatrist:
- Pain that limits the ability to move or function
- Spasticity that makes a limb hard to move
- Falls
- Loss of normal bowel and bladder function

WHAT PRECAUTIONS SHOULD BE TAKEN?

When talking to a physiatrist, listen to everything suggested, but also guide the doctor toward what you specifically want to accomplish. For instance, saying, "I want to be able to open my hand" is more effective than "I want to move better."

*   *   *

USING THE WISDOM OF ATHLETES

One group of people knows the secrets of improving physical movement more than any other: athletes. The definition of athletes is broadened here, to anyone who uses the full range of physical movement in their career or as their passion. By this definition, dancers, martial artists, acrobats, Yoga instructors, and others would be included. The secrets of recovery from stroke are hidden in the tens of thousands of years of developments within these disciplines. There is little that is essential in the development and progress of athletes that is not essential to the process of recovery from stroke.

Here is a list of things athletes and stroke survivors have in common:
- Both want and need to move better.
- Both benefit from weight training.
- Both benefit from cardiovascular training.
- Both use neuroplasticity ("rewiring" of the brain) to move better.
- Both benefit from working on the exact skill they're interested in (known as **task-specific training**).
- Both benefit from **massed practice** (defined as hours of practice at a time).
- Neither of them gains from belief in a **plateau**.
- Both need to measure progress to improve.
- Both benefit from goal setting.
- Both benefit from **mental practice**.
- Both need coaching.
- Both know that the more they challenge themselves, the more progress they will see.
- Both benefit from an upward spiral of success. Successful completion of one goal leads to new challenges and new successes.
- Both benefit from training on the edge of their current ability.

HOW IS IT DONE?

Much of what applies to athletic training is useful to the recovery of stroke survivors because stroke survivors and athletes share the same goal: to get better. The stakes may be higher for stroke survivors but the quest is the same. Learn from athletes; learn from their training techniques and be inspired by their extraordinary level of commitment.

Here are some of the examples of the elements of athletic training covered in this book:

- **Cardiovascular** exercise (see The Ultimate Stroke-Recovery Drug, page 13)
- Weight training (see Weight Up!, page 107)
- **Mental practice** (see Imagine It!, page 78)
- Stretching (see Stretch Out, page 54)
- Development of a training plan (see Plan Your Work and Work Your Plan, page 2)
- Extraordinarily dedicated and hard work

- Measurement of progress (see Measuring Progress, page 16)
- Not accepting plateau as anything but temporary (see Say No to Plateau, page 4)
- A healthy diet (see Eat to Recover, page 125) and sleep (see Fight Fatigue, page 162) to improve
- The use of the **neuroplastic** process to turn their brains into movement machines (see Use Your Fantastic Plastic Brain, page 6)

It is important to understand the kinship between you and the training athlete. When you need direction, inspiration, or a window on how to train, you can look to athletes for guidance. Much of what is known about the development of muscle, **cardiovascular** strength, coordination, balance, and every other aspect of human movement is thanks to the trial-and-error experimentation by athletes over thousands of years.

Many of the magazine articles, research articles, and books on athletic achievement and training can be used to direct recovery from stroke. As the quest for recovery from stroke continues, you can use the essential elements of athletic training in your recovery. Also, athletes are role models of dedicated training. If an athlete were to focus on recovery, she would dream about recovery and plan her days around therapy.

WHAT PRECAUTIONS SHOULD BE TAKEN?

Athletes are athletes and stroke survivors are not. While the analogy has been made here to educate and motivate, it is not intended to encourage unhealthy risk taking. Consult your doctor and physical or occupational therapist prior to superimposing athletic training on your personal training regimen. ”

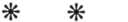

THE ULTIMATE STROKE RECOVERY DRUG

Doctors say it all the time: "If exercise were a pill it would be the most prescribed drug in the world." Being in shape is vital to the recovery process after a stroke. Recovery takes energy. **Neuroplasticity** takes energy.

It takes much more energy for stroke survivors to do everyday tasks. Stroke survivors have, on average, half the amount of cardiovascular strength as age-matched, non-stroke survivors who are out of shape. Many daily activities, most notably walking, take twice the amount energy compared to people who've not had a stroke. Also, the natural aging process reduces muscle strength, heart and blood vessel health, and lung function. For all these reasons it is important to develop a commitment to exercise. Research strongly shows that cardiovascular exercise like walking, and strength training, increases a stroke survivor's chance of becoming more functional. In fact, cardio work (walking, swimming, etc.) and muscle work (weight training) are probably the single most important elements of stroke recovery. Exercise is essential in order to store energy to use in the recovery effort.

Here are some reasons that that an exercise program should include both cardio exercise and strength-training exercises:

- After stroke, you tend to get less of a natural cardio workout in your everyday life. Because walking, bicycling, jogging, etc., are limited after the stroke, you do them less. You should try to counteract this reduction in everyday cardio exercise by doing safe and challenging planned exercises.
- Stroke survivors need more cardiovascular strength than other folks their age because a stroke causes many activities, especially walking, to require more energy because movement is less efficient.
- There is more chance of a stroke survivor having a second stroke than there is for people having a first stroke. Maintaining strong muscles and healthy heart and blood vessels are vital to reducing the risk of another stroke.
- Strength training, done correctly, can increase mobility (i.e., walking, wheelchair mobility) and make transfers easier (lying to sitting, sitting to standing, etc.).
- Rehabilitation efforts toward stroke recovery require stamina. Short-term bursts, as well as day-long amounts of energy are required. Motivation means little when you've exhausted your energy and are too tired to try.
- Weight gain increases the risk of diabetes and blood vessel and heart disease. Muscles burn calories, even at rest. This is not true of other forms of tissue. For example, fat burns no energy (calories). Main-

taining strong muscles and healthy heart and blood vessels is vital in maintaining optimal weight.

- As crazy as it may sound, exercise actually increases energy levels.
- Exercise can increase the amount and quality of sleep you get. The better the sleep, the more energy you can put toward recovery.

HOW IS IT DONE?

Have a physical or occupational therapist design a cardiovascular workout that will be challenging and safe. Let the therapist know, up front, that you want an exercise program that can eventually be done safely at home. A physical therapist will be able to provide leg weight-training exercises that will benefit your walking and overall fitness. For the arm, a similar process should happen with an occupational therapist. Ask for an at-home exercise program that

- Will be safe
- Has progression built in so that the workout remains challenging over the long haul
- Challenges your muscles and your cardiovascular systems

Therapists should be able to develop an at-home program with one to three visits. The therapist calls this sort of at-home therapy, a **home exercise program** (HEP) (see page 100).

Being in shape is essential to recovery and has been a lifestyle choice for many folks after their stroke. Going to the gym, doing physical work (i.e., gardening, housecleaning), and walking instead of driving are all choices that can get folks into better shape. The more strength that can be stored, the more energy can be directed toward recovery. This extra energy can propel an upward spiral of more energy and more strength, which can lead to more recovery, more effort toward exercise, and so on.

Exercise should not necessarily focus totally on the affected ("bad") side. Stroke survivors can benefit from exercising all four limbs, developing cardiovascular endurance, balance, strength, and agility.

WHAT PRECAUTIONS SHOULD BE TAKEN?

There are risk factors with every form of exercise, so consult your doctor prior to changing or starting a new exercise program. Your doctor and a therapist trained in stroke therapy will be able to direct you to the correct mix of exercises. These exercises will be designed to be safe and specifically designed for you, to promote your recovery. Make sure that the exercises are stroke specific. Many "exercise professionals" are not qualified to develop an exercise program for the specialized needs of stroke survivors. Stroke survivors need therapists to develop an exercise program that will help with the specific needs required for stroke recovery. And, above all, therapists can design programs that are safe.

❋   ❋   ❋

MEASURING PROGRESS

How do you know if you are recovering? How do you know if you've achieved one of your goals? Some aspects of recovery from stroke are easy to measure. The first time you walk, climbs stairs, or write your name, are all milestones that should be celebrated. These examples are easy to observe and identify. "I walked for the first time today!" Everyone understands what happened in this case and is willing to give kudos for the accomplishment. Medical staff, therapists, family members, and friends are there to thrill at the gains made. As recovery continues, attaining goals will generally prove more subtle and harder for most folks to see. Walking a little bit faster may mean you can cross the street safely, but it may not be seen by the world as significant. This is one of the reasons that measuring progress is so important. Accurate measurement of progress will reveal small but important gains. Small incremental steps toward recovery may mean:

- The difference between independence and dependence
- The difference between progress toward recovery and ending progress completely
- The beginning of new skills, which allow for new challenges, which in turn allow for new gains, and so on

You may be progressing greatly, but you don't see it. It is hard to accurately remember where you were a week, or a month, or a year ago. There is a tendency to make judgments on where you were yesterday. Maybe yesterday was a really good day and you made great progress. Maybe today is a really bad day and you actually got a little...worse. Many folks will give up, believing they have had a bad day, or a series of bad days. "I'm not getting better, so why should I keep this up?" It may be that you are simply unable to see progress because the day-to-day changes are too small to detect. Relying on memory makes you unable "see the forest through the trees." Recovery should be judged by what happens over an extended arc of time. It's like the stock market. You would put yourself through a lot of stress (and some people do!) with day-by-day details of how your stocks are doing. Investors in the stock market know that what is important is the overall upward trend. Both stocks and stroke recovery involve collecting short-term information in order to see long-term trends.

Any person trying to learn any new skill has benchmarks that he feels he has to meet or exceed. Athletes use clocked speed, amount of weight lifted, batting average, and other measures to determine progress. Musicians have recitals as well as the ability to play new chords, songs, or pieces. The need to measure progress is just as great for stroke survivors. Here are some facts about measuring the progress of your recovery:

- Effective interventions can help you recover faster than you ever imagined.
- If your measurements *do* show progress, you will be more motivated to continue.
- Honestly and accurately gauging *lack* of progress is an essential part of your recovery effort as well. Interventions that are not effective are a waste of time, money, and effort.
- Measuring progress will reveal gains (or losses) that you might not otherwise see.
- Measuring progress will help you determine if your mix of techniques, exercises, modalities, etc., is working.
- In short, measuring progress will determine what is working—and what is not.

If a treatment, modality, exercise, or technique is working, keep it. But if something is not working it should be ruthlessly pitched. The key is accurately measuring the effectiveness of your overall recovery strategy. Because all interventions affect each other, you are not really evaluating individual interventions. Rather, you are measuring your current mix of interventions.

HOW IS IT DONE?

Without accurate data, assumptions about recovery are nothing more than guessing. Imagine a researcher scratching his head and saying, "Boy, I dunno. I *think* they're getting better." It would certainly lack merit!

You do not need complicated data collection tools and a lot of computing power to measure progress. There are easy ways of measuring progress that are inexpensive and accurate. No matter what is measured or how it is measured, recording, either through notes (i.e., "I walked three blocks today in 5 minutes") or by other methods (i.e., viewing videotape of your walking) will allow you to accurately compare the past to the present. In short, measurement can be done efficiently, simply, and with modest expertise and little equipment.

Here are some ways to measure progress that take little training and equipment:

- *Timing how quickly something can be done*: From walking a specific distance, to saying a sentence, everything can be timed. Timing can be of two speeds; the fastest possible and "self-selected" speed. Self-selected speed is the speed that is comfortable and natural. Self-selected speeds have the advantage of more accurately assessing speed of an activity in real-world, normal, and natural circumstances. Timing the fastest possible speed has the advantage of providing a more apples-to-apples comparison.
- *Timing how long something can be done*: The length of time that an activity can be performed can reveal valuable information about endurance. For instance, the ability to propel a wheelchair for 4 consecutive minutes today is better than 2 minutes last week.
- *Observation as evaluation*: Using a mirror can provide valuable, real-time feedback as to the nature of the quality of movement. This sort of measurement is inherently subjective, but can reveal valuable insight into strengths and deficits.
- *Videotaping different tasks*: Video can provide a viewable historical account of progress.

- *Audio- or videotaping speech*: Progress toward improving speech can be evaluated with an audio recording. Videotaping speech has the advantage of seeing the quality of movement of the mouth. Sometimes, however, it is better to not view the speech, but rather evaluate speech only by the quality of the sound. This is because while mouth movements may not be pretty, "ugly" movement may produce the best speech. This is true in expressive aphasia (difficulty speaking) that involves dysarthria. Dysarthria is when the muscles of the mouth don't work well because of damage to the area of the brain that moves the mouth.
- *Counting repetitions*: The number of a particular exercise performed can indicate muscle strength and endurance.
- *Measuring distance*: Measuring the distance walked is the most obvious example, but there are other aspects of recovery that can be assessed by measuring distance. For instance, the distance reached across a table with the hand or the length of a step can also measure progress.
- *Take blood pressure and pulse*: Blood pressure and pulse are indicators of cardiovascular health. They are also important indicators of the progress of recovery. Decreased blood pressure and resting heart rate (pulse) are seen as positive health indicators. This is not always the case, however. If there is a jump in heart rate and blood pressure, either higher or lower, consult you doctor. Cardiovascular health is essential for stroke survivors because the stroke itself is an indication of imperfect cardiovascular health. Stroke, whether a bleed (**hemorrhagic**) or block (**ischemic**) is a (very) significant vascular event. See page 62 "Five Tests You Should Do" for more information about testing pulse and blood pressure.

"When and how often should I measure progress?" you may ask. The more the better is the general rule. The important thing is to be constant and consistent in measuring and recording your data. Once you have collected your information, write it down in a logbook or calendar. For instance, you may write down the time it takes to walk around a quarter-mile track. Every time you make the walk, write down the time. Your measurement will show less and less time to make the quarter-mile walk. This decrease in time may continue for months. At some point, your times will not improve, unless you change the way you train. Recovery options that involve **massed**

practice should be evaluated in the short term (1-3 weeks). These options tend to ask for a lot of intense short-term effort. Change should be measurable in the first couple of weeks. Other activities, like those that involve increasing stamina and muscle strength, take longer to show results.

WHAT PRECAUTIONS SHOULD BE TAKEN?

Measurement works to modify behavior because most people try to beat their previous best. Measurement represents you competing against yourself. Any time there is a competition, there is going to be the tendency to reach for the edge of your ability. This striving can put you in danger. An example would be, "I'm going to beat my best time for walking around the block." This aggressive attempt could lead to less safety awareness—which could lead to a fall. Be aware of your own limitations.

Recovery Hints and Tricks

CHALLENGE EQUALS RECOVERY

Stroke makes movement difficult. Overcoming the difficulty creates a productive struggle that propels recovery. If you eliminate the difficulty, you will not progress toward recovery. This is true with any growth in any aspect of your life: the challenge itself cultivates growth.

There is a tendency for some stroke survivors to halt their own progress by only working on what they can. For instance, with their doctor's blessing, they may go to the gym and do weight training, an action with positive intentions. Once at the gym, however, they work with the muscles that they can control with ease, while ignoring the muscles that pose more of a challenge. All muscles should be strengthened, including the ones that are cooperating. But emphasis should be placed on muscles that are not easy to flex and on movements that provide the most challenge. Challenge is the essence of recovery. To shy away from the challenges inherent in recovery is to shy away from recovery itself.

Stroke survivors will benefit if they concentrate on what they can't do, not what they can. For instance, if you can make a fist but find it hard to open the fisted hand, then work on opening it. The ability to make a fist needs little encouragement. But the ability to open the hand is just as important and, since it is more of a challenge, opening the hand requires more attention. "If I can't open my hand, then what's the use of trying? It won't open!" The movement you are trying to accomplish may need attention. If a hand is fisted and hard to open there are suggestions throughout this book (i.e., injectable muscle relaxants, electrical stimulation) to aid in its opening. The point is not to ignore the movements that are difficult and challenging. Embrace them. Ironically, overcoming the challenges left in the wake of a stroke is the best way to recover from stroke! If you eliminate the difficulty and only do what you are now able, you would never relearn how to move better. Challenge drives **neuroplasticity**. Neuroplasticity drives recovery.

HOW IS IT DONE?

Make an honest and accurate account of your strengths and weakness. List the things that need work, and make that list one of the tools for navigating toward recovery. Focus recovery efforts on actions that you have real problems performing rather than accentuating those abilities that are near perfect. Recovery from stroke involves making an honest assessment and a constant reassessment of what needs work and what does not. It is simply a matter of priorities. Fortunately, areas of relative deficit, much more than areas of relative strength, provide greater potential for improvement and recovery. Athletes know this. Athletes launch themselves headlong into any challenge that stands between them and winning. Your recovery will accelerate if you honor the challenges that make up the recovery process.

WHAT PRECAUTIONS SHOULD BE TAKEN?

Recovery from stroke is hard work. Devoting effort to movements and tasks that are difficult and challenging takes a lot of energy, concentration, and focus. Sometimes the challenge is so difficult that it takes many attempts before the movement or task is accomplished. While this may be safe for some tasks (i.e., attempting to open the hand), it may be dangerous for other tasks (i.e., attempting to walk). Every challenge needs to be undertaken with safety in mind because nothing stops recovery like an injury.

*   *   *

USE WHAT YOU HAVE

After stroke, survivors typically move in what is called "synergistic movement." Synergistic movement does not allow the joints of the limbs on the "bad" side move independently. For instance, if a stroke survivor tries to bring her hand forward, her elbow comes up to shoulder height, the elbow bends, and the shoulder joint elevates. All these movements are said to be linked. You can't do one movement without doing a whole bunch of other unnecessary movements. This is the way stroke survivors naturally move, and there is nothing wrong with it. As recovery progresses, these movements will become "unlinked" and individual joints will begin to move more normally. Unfortunately there is a belief on the part of many therapists that this sort of movement is "bad" movement and should never be done. Therapists believe that using this type of movement will somehow be learned so well that it can't be unlearned...like a bad habit. This thinking is as misguided as believing that, because babies fall a lot as they learn to walk, they will only learn how to fall and never learn to walk!

HOW IS IT DONE?

Many therapists feel the need to intervene, often with a hands-on approach, to make sure stroke survivors are moving correctly. But there are two problems with this approach:

1. Your efforts toward recovery should be **patient driven**. This means that you are responsible for your own recovery. If it is essential that a therapist be involved to ensure correct movement, then the recovery process is taken out of the hands of the stroke survivor. There is simply not enough time (nor money!) if your recovery effort depends on having therapists by your side during the entire recovery process. Therapists are essential at different times during the recovery process. But much of your recovery is going to happen between periods of clinical therapy. After the stroke, therapy is paid for by insurance and Medicare for approximately a few months. Once therapy ends, it is not the beginning of the end of your recovery, just the end of the beginning. There is still much work to do. And you will have to do that work without the luxury of having anyone there to remind you of the "right way" to move.

2. Relearning to move after stroke is like learning any new skill you've learned in your life. The process of trial and error is essential to learning how to move correctly. Mistakes allow for corrections, and corrections lead to greater recovery. Use what movement is available, no matter how unwieldy!

I have a saying, "**massed practice** beats **mass synergies**." Mass synergy is the term used to describe the movements that are always linked together (massed) after stroke. This is the movement that many therapists see as unwanted and to be discouraged. Research has shown that repeated practice, known as repetitive massed practice, can overcome these mass synergies. If done correctly and with large amounts of motivation and dedication, diligent practice allows the lack of coordination, linked movements, and awkwardness to melt away.

WHAT PRECAUTIONS SHOULD BE TAKEN?

Usage of synergistic movement (the awkward movement after stroke) is not dangerous and will not ingrain those movements. Use the movement you have!

✳   ✳   ✳

TRAIN WELL ON A TREADMILL

A treadmill is an effective recovery tool for folks who have had a stroke... as long as it is safe. Researchers have found that treadmill training can improve walking quality and increase walking speed. Research has shown that increased walking speed has a positive effect on:

- Cardiovascular fitness (important in reducing risk of another stroke)
- Muscle strength (important for overall fitness and maintaining optimal weight)
- Balance (important in reducing the risk of falls)
- Coordination (important in reducing the amount of energy it takes to walk, which gives you the ability to walk faster and for longer distances)

Treadmill training can also boost confidence in everyday walking around the house and around the community.

Treadmills have the advantage of:

- Providing a safe, straight, flat, and never-ending path on which to walk
- Providing handles that offer endless parallel bars (the bars that stroke survivors hold on to while taking their first steps after stroke)
- Allowing long-distance walking in comfortable indoor settings
- Providing gradation of speed and incline (steepness)

- Allowing for detailed measurement of progress (usually provided as a digital readout about distance and speed on the treadmill's dashboard)

HOW IS IT DONE?

The first step (forgive the pun) is to consider the safety issues involved in treadmill training given your level of walking ability. This question can be answered by a single visit to a physical therapist, who will evaluate safety issues. The therapist will review how to safely step on and off a treadmill, as well as evaluate what speed is safe and challenging, given your fitness level. This therapy session should also include information on how to make treadmill training challenging as your walking improves. The physical therapist will review how and when to increase speed, distance, and incline as time goes on.

The next step is buying a treadmill, and they can be expensive. Alternatively, consider joining a gym (Space to Focus—The Community Gym, page 104) that has treadmills. The money you save on the treadmill purchase can be put toward a gym membership. On the other hand, there are several advantages to having the treadmill in your home:

- The visual reminder of having the piece of equipment in your home
- The convenience. No travel, no traffic, no time lost
- You control the environment, including the music
- You can exercise whenever you are in the mood

A few hundred dollars can provide all the features you'll need. Look for a treadmill that has:

- A motorized walking surface with at least 1.5 horsepower
- The ability to provide an incline (the ability for the walking surface to lift, as if you're walking uphill). Stroke survivors often have "drop foot," which is an inability to lift the foot at the ankle. Increasing the incline of the walking surface increases the challenge to the foot to lift at the ankle. This will develop coordination and strength in the muscles that lift the foot.
- Handrails that are both comfortable and that you can grasp quickly if needed
- An auto shut-off button that allows you to shut off the treadmill quickly. Look for treadmills that have a tethered cord that you at-

tach to your clothes, which automatically shuts off the treadmill if
you lose your balance.
* Easy-to-read digital numbers

Always try out the treadmill before you buy it. Wear the same clothes
and shoes you would normally use on the treadmill.

The question of where to place a treadmill requires some consideration.
There are the considerations of space and where in your home is appropriate
to do the hard work of improving your walking. Before you buy a treadmill,
measure the length, width, and height of the space where you expect to
place it. There is also the question of distractions. If you put a treadmill in
an area where there is a TV, radio, or other distractions, is this a good thing
or a bad thing? Some therapists believe that stroke survivors should focus
only on their walking. Other therapists believe that, since real-world walking
involves a variety of distractions (i.e., TV, conversations, phone, traffic noise,
etc.) the training should involve similar distractions.

If your stroke caused a limp, treadmill walking will not necessarily decrease it, if you do not try to look at and attempt to correct the quality of
gait. During walking you have limited visual feedback because you see your
walking from above, looking down toward your feet. You can better evaluate
your walking by having a mirror at the end of a treadmill and walking "toward" the mirror.

WHAT PRECAUTIONS SHOULD BE TAKEN?

Treadmills are relatively safe for some stroke survivors, but even for
stroke survivors who walk well, treadmills have the potential to injure. The
best way to determine the safety of treadmill walking for a particular stroke
survivor is to have a quick visit with a physical therapist and let his expertise
guide you. Precautions should be taken to ensure the proper use of the machine and that the treadmill is used within appropriate cardiovascular limits.
Those who use **assistive devices** such as canes and walkers need to take special care. Treadmills are like moving sidewalks that have an electrical motor,
which moves the floor belt in the direction opposite of the direction walked.
This fact provides inherent risks. For instance, if the stroke survivor stops
walking, the treadmill will keep him moving backward. This is why it is
important for treadmills to have a tethering system, so that if the person

walking is carried backward by the machine, the treadmill will stop. This failsafe may be appropriate for some stroke survivors.

Before you get on any treadmill, make sure you know how to slow it down, speed it up, and the location of the emergency-off button. Understanding how to safely and appropriately operate the treadmill that you use will allow for a safe, productive, and enjoyable experience.

✳   ✳   ✳

MIRRORS REFLECT RECOVERY

As babies learn how to move (i.e., crawling, walking, moving hands and fingers), the experience is new, and much of this learning is a process of trial and error. Every movement is new and interesting, and the infant is naturally drawn to the effort because of the sheer fun of practicing. Children and adults learn new movements in much the same way. However, the way people learn how to move as infants, children, and adults is different from learning how to move *after* stroke, because after a stroke, it is *relearning*. Rehabilitation from stroke involves relearning movements that, prior to the stroke, you did perfectly. Your memory (and observing the unaffected side of your body) provides a clear image of what the movement looked and felt like. But many stroke survivors have problems accurately feeling where their limbs are in space (**proprioception**) and have a decreased sense of touch, pressure, and temperature. The question becomes, how can you relearn how to move when you can't feel how you're moving?

An easy way to determine if movement is being accomplished correctly is to use a mirror. If you walk toward a mirror, you allow yourself instant feedback about the symmetry (evenness) of the two lower limbs during gait (see Train Well on a Treadmill, page 25). Mirrors can also be used to evaluate the coordination, potential strength, and health of the entire affected side, including upper and lower extremities and the trunk.

Many stroke survivors refuse to look at the stroke-affected arm and hand. Even after they are reminded to look at the hand they often will only glance at it as if it holds little interest to them. This is especially true in folks who are

apraxic (an inability to accurately plan movements). *Once a mirror is introduced, there is often a fascination by survivors with movement on the "bad" side.* This fascination can provide a renewed focus on their quality of movement.

HOW IS IT DONE?

Mirrors are especially important in helping stroke survivors evaluate themselves because stroke causes an imbalance between the "good" and "bad" sides. This lack of balance between the limbs includes differences in strength, coordination, feeling, and muscle size. This causes the stroke survivors to often use only the "good" arm and leg because it makes life easier. And, remember, the less you use the "bad" limbs, the more the part of the brain involved in that movement will shrink. Use it or lose it was never truer.

Meanwhile the part of the brain that controls the unaffected limbs will improve because you are using that part of the brain more. The "good" limbs get better and better, while the affected limbs get worse and worse. The unaffected upper extremity may now be asked to write, do one-handed shoe tying, or be used in feeding. Using only the "good side" limbs to do activities of daily living is called **compensatory movement**. Compensatory movement promotes coordination in the unaffected limb while also promoting less coordination in the "bad" limb. The survivor should focus on the quality of the movement of the affected limb, and this is where mirrors help. When you look in the mirror, do both arms and hands have the same quality of movement? How are they moving differently? What can be done to make the movements more symmetrical? While doing something with both hands and arms that involve different but cooperative movements (like dealing cards or unscrewing a cap), look closely for quality movement from the affected arm and hand. Make every effort to have the "bad" side limbs copy how the "good" side moves.

Many stroke survivors have an inability to judge where their limbs are in space if they are not looking directly at them. Again, the feel of where the limb is in space, even with the eyes closed, is called **proprioception**. Proprioception is often lost on the affected side after a stroke. Mirrors can help evaluate if proprioception is, or is not, intact. Try this experiment:

- Face a mirror so you can see your arms and hands.
- Close your eyes.

- Have someone move the "bad" arm and hand into a position and hold you in that position.
- Keeping your eyes closed, move the "good" arm and hand to match the position of the "bad" limb.
- Open your eyes.

Look at yourself moving in front of a mirror. When the limb is seen in the mirror, does it feel like where it actually is? Are both limbs in the same position? Some neurologists (doctors who deal with the nerves, brain, and the spinal cord) believe that stroke survivors may be able relearn proprioception by "rewiring" their brains (**neuroplasticity**). The process of relearning proprioception is done using the same principles of neuroplasticity that are used to relearn movement. Constant visual feedback will begin to retrain the brain to remember how movements feel. This feedback can be provided by doing anything from weight training to **repetitive practice** while facing a mirror.

Mirrors can also be used to judge symmetry in the arms and legs. Is the arm or leg affected by the stroke the same size as the unaffected limb? Are the limbs the same color? Do they have the same amount of hair? Does one look swollen compared to the other? All of these observations can give you insight into the way your body is recovering. Looking for balance between the left and right limbs and other observations in the mirror is probably best done with clothing that reveals as much skin surface area as possible.

WHAT PRECAUTIONS SHOULD BE TAKEN?

Inform your doctor about any changes that you observe that seem out of the ordinary. Decreased muscle bulk on the affected side is to be expected. Swelling, loss of hair, or change in skin color, however, may indicate something more serious.

✳   ✳   ✳

STICK TO THE TASK

There is a reason that athletes and musicians tend to excel at what they do: they practice a lot! What movements do athletes and musicians practice?

They practice the exact movements, or parts of the movements that they will perform during the game or concert. This is called **task-specific training**. Athletes and musicians are great role models for stroke survivors because they demonstrate the value of dedicated practice. There are other people, people you may see working every day, who are experts in particular movements. From typing to carpet weaving and from knitting to working on an assembly line, there are many examples of task-specific training. The folks who work in these jobs know that the more they practice, the better they will become.

You may wonder why you should try doing things that you know you either can't do or won't do well. Research has shown that task-specific practice is the best way to improve upon a given task. Remember, movements done with the arm and legs change the way the brain is wired. When you practice the specific task that you want to recover, you rewire the brain to be better at that task.

HOW IS IT DONE?

When doing task-specific training it is essential to try activities that you really care about. The more cherished the task, the more focus will be brought to the training and the more neuroplastic rewiring will occur. The level of importance of a task can be expressed as this continuum:

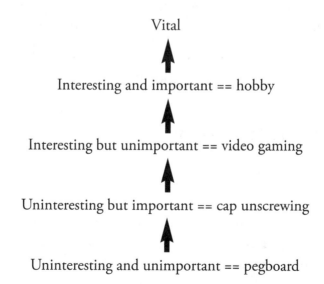

Vital

↑

Interesting and important == hobby

↑

Interesting but unimportant == video gaming

↑

Uninteresting but important == cap unscrewing

↑

Uninteresting and unimportant == pegboard

For example, consider George, a stroke survivor who wants to get back to playing the game of golf, which he loves. He knows he'll never play golf again, so he does not think to mention it to his therapist. George is unable to turn his forearm so his palm faces up. His therapist has him flip cards to develop this movement. George could care less and feels like he's spending too much time flipping cards. The therapist then has him play a video game where he has to manipulate a joystick by turning his hand palm-up and palm-down. He finds the game interesting for a while, and then gets bored. The therapist has George pretend to shave with a razor handle with no blade. George finds the task important. He does have to shave, but then again, he could do it with his "good" hand. Then the therapist suggests he start putting a golf ball. At first George refuses. "I'd rather remember my game the way it was." The therapist is surprised to hear that George is a golfer, and encourages him to try. George is told to try to putt one-handed with his affected hand, trying to turn his forearm so he can putt the ball straight. George goes home with his forearm aching. "That was fun!" he says. He doesn't even wait for the next therapy session. He goes to a sporting goods shop that evening and buys an electric ball return. He starts to imagine returning to golf!

WHAT PRECAUTIONS SHOULD BE TAKEN?

Task-specific practice is tiring because the motivation to perform the activity is high. Fatigue can lead to accidents. Ask your doctor and/or therapist if the chosen task is appropriate to further your recovery, and safe.

*　*　*

LET RECOVERY FLOW

Everybody is most motivated by the activities they love. There is a natural tendency to focus on, practice, and pursue activities you love to do. When the stroke survivor works on things that she is passionate about, it is no longer work, rehabilitation, or exercise. Recovery becomes play. Athletes talk about being "in flow." Being in flow is when you are so immersed in an activity that you lose track of time. When an athlete is in flow, all the problems in his life melt away and all that is left is his sport. You can use flow in recovery. Being in the flow of recovery:

- Eliminates self-doubt and self-consciousness
- Allows you to focus on recovery on an instinctive level
- Allows you to focus on nothing but recovery
- Makes recovery enjoyable
- Makes time seem to stand still
- Reduces any aches and pains associated with recovery
- Makes recovery addictive because the feeling of being in flow is addictive

HOW IS IT DONE?

One of the most important concepts in stroke recovery is this: **necessity drives recovery**. Define what is essential to your:

- Identity (work, family)
- Passions (hobbies, your art, sports)
- Happiness (playing with grandchildren, attending church)
- Life (cooking, cleaning, grooming)
- Independence (walking)

Walking is a great example of "necessity drives recovery." Everyone who has a stroke knows the importance of walking. Work to recover everything that you really want, the same way you relearned walking. Identify what is most important to you, and use those things to drive your recovery. If you are working toward goals that you really care about, your effort toward recovery is magnified. Research studies have shown that when stroke survivors focus on *meaningful* activities they get better, faster. "Meaningful" suggests an emotional content to what is being practiced. Consider someone who played drums before his or her stroke. Using the act of drumming to help recovery makes his or her efforts meaningful. A nondrummer who uses drumming for recovery may find the practice *interesting*. But because there is no emotional attachment to drums, he won't see the practice as *meaningful*.

Focusing on "necessity drives recovery" has the advantage of focusing recovery efforts on tasks that you care about. Pick tasks that are meaningful to you. Finding the tasks that you are passionate about, that you can't live without, or that help you with independence. Choosing important tasks will help recovery in a way that nothing else can. The athlete knows what causes him to be in flow. Deciding what is essential to you is the first step to recovering in flow. For instance, eating may be an important goal. But it may be faster and easier to eat with the unaffected hand, so what is the motivation? Now change the goal to cooking using the affected arm and hand. If cooking is meaningful to you then you are automatically motivated to use the bad arm and hand. Your passion for cooking will propel you to greater levels of recovery.

Therapy in a clinic may be effective but not necessarily motivating. Consider playing catch as an example. Therapists often play games of catch with stroke survivors in order to challenge balance, arm movement, and reaction time. This sort of exercise may be fun, and it may indeed help recovery. But catch may not hold any importance to the stroke survivor. Therapists use treatments to help make you safer and more functional. But once you return home, motivation may be lost if you are not working on a meaningful goal. The more important the activity is to you, the more motivated you will be. And the more motivated you are, the more recovery you'll get. **Necessity drives recovery**. Practicing what you really care about can provide motivation for other tasks that you may find boring. For instance, you may find treadmill walking boring and tedious. But if you are a golfer and treadmill walking follows the yardage of a favorite golf course (a typical golf course involves about five miles of walking!) then you will be more motivated to train on a treadmill.

Once the activity is achievable and safe, the activity itself can be used to drive recovery. Consider walking. If you are a walking enthusiast, then walking is the meaningful goal even before you regained the ability to walk. Once the ability to walk is gained, the act of walking can be safely used to improve your walking. And more walking leads to increased speed and distance, provides better coordination of gait, increases cardiovascular health, and an upward spiral of recovery is set.

Sometimes doing the activity is impossible because you just don't have enough strength and coordination. So you take the small steps necessary toward building strength and coordination. Even when you are taking the small steps toward the meaningful activity, the activity should always be in view. This may involve having the tools of that activity visible. Even if you are unable to achieve any part of the activity right now, the meaningful goal should be the guiding light as you move toward that goal.

WHAT PRECAUTIONS SHOULD BE TAKEN?

Incorporating activities that you find meaningful into the process of rehabilitation is a positive move, as long as those activities are safe. If you loved to mountain climb prior to the stroke, then pursuit of that particular passion probably won't be safe—in the short run at least! Attempt cherished activities with common sense. The stroke survivor should stay within his or her skill level and make safety the number-one priority.

✳   ✳   ✳

THE RECOVERY CALENDAR

Appointment calendars keep people organized and on schedule. Important appointments, including doctors' appointments, business appointments, and meetings are all noted. Your recovery efforts deserve a calendar, too. The recovery calendar will help you stay on schedule, and the act of crossing off the items will be partial reward for all the hard work you've done. Keeping a recovery calendar is an easy way to stay motivated and focused. The calendar itself is a reminder to work toward recovery. Also, a calendar helps you evaluate the effectiveness of you recovery effort, the progress you've made, and the goals you wish to achieve. A workout calendar is an essential part of the overall recovery plan.

A calendar dedicated to recovery will:

- Keep track of successes and failures
- Help establish what works and what does not
- Help spot positive and negative trends in the quest toward recovery
- Help separate effective therapies from lemons
- Help measure progress by providing an accessible and detailed account of the arc of recovery. For instance, you may see that the

longest walk last month was 20 yards and the longest walk this week
was twice that amount.

- Record progress, which is essential to defining and achieving goals
- Help increase adherence to goals
- Add to the sense of accomplishment as goals are met
- Provide an accurate record on which to look back
- Provide valuable information to doctors and therapists as they help
  you plan your recovery

A calendar can also be used to set new goals. Calendars allow you to
look back and see what you've accomplished, but you can also set new goals
for the future. For instance, if in April you walked 100 yards in a single
walk, you might be able to project that you can walk 150 yards by
June 15th. You can then anticipate and train toward specific projected goals.

HOW IS IT DONE?

Workout calendars are commercially available in bookstores, as down-
loads from the Internet, or one can be made using personal computer word-
processing programs. A recovery calendar only needs three elements:

1. A row for dates
2. A column for the interventions, exercises, or modalities
3. Columns and rows of boxes to input appropriate statistics

An example of a recovery calendar follows the next section. *Do not consider this example as a suggested course of interventions.*

Use a pencil when filling out your calendar. This will give you the ability
to correct mistakes and change future goals.

WHAT PRECAUTIONS SHOULD BE TAKEN?

There are no specific precautions that should be taken for the actual calendar. Discuss daily recovery activities with your doctor. Please note that the
calendar example provided (see Table on page 37) is not a representation of
any existing calendar. Do not consider the example as a suggested course of
interventions.

✳   ✳   ✳

Week begin 5/12/08 / Week end 5/18/08	Mon	Tues	Wed	Thurs	Fri.	Sat.	Sun.
	12	13	14	15	16	17	18
Walking	Around the block x 3	Off	Around the block x 3	Around the block x 4!!	Off	Twice around the block x 3	Off
Elec. stimulation	Wrist and finger ext. (15 m)	Wrist and finger ext. (15 m)	Wrist, muscles feel stiff (0 m)	Wrist and finger ext. (15 m)	Wrist and finger ext. (15 m)	Wrist and finger ext. (15 m)	Off
Mental practice	Throwing a ball sequence	Throwing a ball sequence	Off	Throwing a ball sequence	Throwing a ball sequence	Off	Off
Rhythmic bilateral arm training	Armcycle to fav. Song #1,2&3 (~15 min)	Drumming to "Rockin' '78" Album (~15 min)	Armcycle to fav. Song #1,2 (~10 min)	Armcycle to fav. Song #1,2&3 (~15 min)	Off	Wiping table with towels to 2 songs (~10 min)	Off
Resistance training (legs)	– Squats 3 sets/10 reps 3lb 3x10 – Hip Abduction 3 lb 3x10	– Hip abduction 3lb 3x10 – "Footups" 3lb 3x10	– Knee-ups 2lb 3lb 3x10 – Hip ext w/ band x 5 min	– Hip Abduction 3lb 3x10 – "Footups" 3lb 3x10	– Knee-ups 2lb 3x10 – Hip ext w/ band x 5 min	– Squats 3 sets/10 reps – knee-ups 2lb 3x10	Off
Resistance training (arms)	Band into elbow ext. 3x10	Band press-ups, pulling forearm out 3x10	Band into elbow ext. 3x10	Off	Band press-ups, pulling forearm out 3x10	Band press-ups, pulling forearm out 3x10	Off
Task specific-training	– Putting – throwing a ball both 20 min	– Throwing a ball 20 min	– Putting 20 min	– Throwing a ball 20 min	– Throwing a ball 20 min	Off	Off
Massed practice	– Foot out x 20 min – grasp release x 20 min	– Foot out x 20 min – grasp release x 20 min	– Foot out x 20 min – grasp release x 20 min	Off	– Foot out x 20 min – grasp release x 20 min	– Foot out x 20 min – grasp release x 20 min	Off
Stretching	Many times through day	Many times through day	Many times through day	Many times through day	Many times through day	Many times through day	Many times through day
Pulse, blood pressure	P = 68 BP = 125/83	P = 67 BP = 127/86	P = 62 BP = 121/80	P = 72 BP = 119/84	P = 65 BP = 127/86	P = 67 BP = 122/78	Off

ROADMAP TO RECOVERY

Hypocrites (460-370 BC), the "father of medicine," was the first to describe stroke, transient ischemic attacks (TIA or mini-stroke), and **aphasia**. As the years passed understanding of the concept of stroke increased, but understanding of recovery remained limited. It was not until 2,400 years after Hypocrites that someone developed a way of predicting the step-by-step progression of recovery. Enter Singe Brunnstrom. Brunnstrom, a Swedish Fulbright Scholar and pioneer physical therapist did much of her work in the 1940s and 1950s. She was the first person to accurately describe the predictable pattern of recovery after stroke. She described the process of recovery from total **paralysis**, to the point at which total recovery is achieved. The amazing aspect of Brunnstrom's roadmap to recovery is that it holds up against today's scientific measures. For instance, doctors and therapists can now see, in the images provided by MRI (magnetic resonance imaging), that **Brunnstrom's stages of recovery** correlate well with **neuroplastic** changes in the brain.

SYNERGY

As recovery from stroke progresses, the limbs begin to move under the control of the brain. But the limbs tend to move in unusual ways. Sometimes the limb cannot make any one movement without making a whole series of unnecessary movements. Typical movement after stroke, where everything in the limb moves at once—even though you don't want it to—is called **synergistic movement** or simply **synergy**.

One example might involve a stroke survivor who attempts to bend her elbow but who cannot bend *only* her elbow. If she tries to bend only her elbow a whole bunch of other movements appear; her shoulder rises and comes back, and at the same time her arm extends from her body. Even her wrist and fingers flex. Synergy makes moving just one part of the arm impossible. All the other parts of the arm join the act. Synergy happens if any part of the limb attempts to move. If you attempt to lift the wrist, the fingers, wrist, elbow, shoulder, and shoulder blade will move. This is true of the lower extremity as well. Movement at the toes, ankle, knee, and hip will cause synergistic movement of the whole limb. Understanding synergy and synergistic movement will help you understand the wealth of wisdom within Brunnstrom's stages of recovery.

HOW IS IT DONE?

Until Brunnstrom described the arc of recovery, there was no agreed-upon roadmap to recovery. Brunnstrom's six stages of recovery provide that roadmap. These six stages also answer many of the questions that you'll have about your recovery including:

- Where you are in the recovery process
- What new skills appear as progress is made
- What challenges are in the existing stage (spastic, synergistic, limp, etc.)
- What you are striving for, and how you'll recognize it when you achieve it

Researchers use tests based on the six stages as an accurate measurement of progress. You can too! As you look back at how far you've come, you'll remember the stages you've overcome. As you continue your progress, you will notice that you are moving through the stages, one by one.

In the first stage, the whole hemiparetic ("bad") side of the body is flaccid, and the sixth stage is total recovery. Here are the six stages.

Stage 1
During the 1st stage, the whole "bad" side is completely limp. The arm, the leg, the torso, the face, including the mouth and tongue are limp.

Stage 2
Spasticity (muscle tightness) starts to creep into the "bad" side of the body. Spasticity is generally considered a good thing because the affected side is no longer limp. Spasticity signals the beginning of messages getting from the nervous system to the limbs. Stage 2 is also when a basic form of synergies appear. There may be some small amount of voluntary movement available, but only within synergy.

Stage 3
During Stage 3, spasticity is at its strongest. Spasticity may become severe during this stage. That is the unfortunate part of Stage 3. The bright side is that you begin to control the synergies. This means

that the limbs can be moved voluntarily as long as the movements are within synergies.

Stage 4

During Stage 4, spasticity begins to decline. In this stage, some movements outside of synergy appear. So, two positive things occur during Stage 4: spasticity declines and synergistic movement begins to decline.

Stage 5

Synergies continue to decline. Folks in Stage 5 enjoy more voluntary control out of synergy. Spasticity continues to decline. Some movements appear normal.

Stage 6

This is the final stage. If this stage is achieved, movements look normal. Spasticity is absent except when fatigued or performing rapid movements. Individual joint movements become possible, and co-ordination approaches normal.

Here is a visual representation of Brunnstrom's stages of recovery from stroke:

No movement

↓

Spasticity is high. Synergies dominate

↓

Movement outside of synergy becomes available

↓

Normal movement, most of the time

WHAT PRECAUTIONS SHOULD BE TAKEN?

Here are some more ideas that relate to the six stages:

- Recovery always moves through the six stages in order. Stages may be brief, but you will go through all of the stages in order. For instance, if you are in Stage 2, you will go through Stage 3 on your way to Stage 4. And you have to go through Stage 4 to get to Stage 5, and so on.

- Even if you do no work and have no therapy, you still might see progress.
- The process of recovery may be quick or slow and may end. This ending of recovery is what is called a **plateau**. (If stroke survivors work hard, plateaus in recovery tend to be temporary periods. These periods can be used to change what you are doing in order to have progress continue. However, stroke survivors sometimes do not, for a variety of reasons, continue to progress.)
- You will see recovery in the joints close to the body (e.g., the shoulder and hip). Recovery will then spread away from the body (e.g., the fingers and toes).
- No two stroke survivors recover in the same way.
- Recovery of the hand is the hardest to predict. The intricate movement of the fingers and the many different motions at the thumb make any predictions almost impossible. The hand is also usually the last part of the body to regain movement.
- Closing of the hand will come back before the ability to open the hand.

*   *   *

RECOVERY WAS SO FAST RIGHT AFTER THE STROKE—WHY DID IT SLOW DOWN?

Six months to 1 year after stroke is called the **acute** period. This is often a period of rapid recovery. Stroke survivors often give credit for this recovery to doctors, therapists, or their own hard work. But there is another important reason recovery is so rapid: much of the recovery results from a reduction of the swelling in the brain.

Nerve cells die during the stroke. This dead area in the brain causes the physical and mental problems that stroke survivors know too well. But there is an area of nerve cells just outside the dead area that survives. The nerve cells in the **penumbra** are alive but are inactive for a while after a stroke.

Some doctors refer to these cells as being "stunned." Doctors work hard to protect these cells because they have the potential to either live or die. The nerve cells that live become active again, usually between a few hours to a few months after stroke. During this period there is often a lot of recovery.

An injury to any part of the body will cause many body systems to come to the aid of the injured area. The same is true after a stroke. After a stroke, there are many chemicals delivered to the site of the area in the brain where the stroke occurred. These chemicals are sent to try to reduce the damage caused by the stroke. Calcium, destructive enzymes, free radicals, nitric oxide, and other chemicals are delivered to the area damaged by the stroke. This result is a "metabolic soup" that "stuns" cells that surround the cells that were killed by the stroke. As the swelling around the area resolves, the chemicals are absorbed back into the body. The stunned cells come back to life. This is the same way any part of the body deals with injury. For example, imagine you bruise the biceps muscle (the big "Popeye" muscle that bends the elbow). The muscle turns black and blue and feels stiff. Below the surface of the skin, many of the body's systems are working to repair the muscle. And just like workers building a house, there is a lot of activity and a lot of mess. As time goes on the activity decreases, the "workers" begin to go home, and the swelling around the injury decreases. This is similar to what happens in a brain that has been injured by stroke. In the short term there is a lot of activity, much of it chemical, directed toward helping the brain heal. As the swelling is reduced, brain cells spring back to life, and movement in the arms and legs improves. Researchers have called this period of rapid recovery "spontaneous recovery" or "natural recovery."

As the swelling goes down, there is rapid recovery. While no part of recovery is easy, the first few months after a stroke often provide a lot of recovery with modest effort. Stroke survivors are encouraged by this period of relatively quick and easy recovery. Hope for full recovery is present. Patients seem to be riding the wave of natural recovery. "Riding a wave" is an accurate metaphor because like a wave, the ride is free, and you can go far, but then it ends. From then on you have to paddle hard. The good news is that dedicated and focused work (when you "paddle hard") can continue to produce results. The point at which natural recovery ends has been commonly viewed as the end of the recovery process. As recovery slows down, physical and occupational therapy ends. Ironically, this is the period when therapists are needed the most, because when natural recovery ends, guidance is essential. But don't blame therapists. Insurance guidelines dictate that once the patient has stopped making measurable progress, therapy must end.

HOW IS IT DONE?

The traditional view has been that recovery ends during the first 6 months to 1 year after stroke. But there is a problem with this viewpoint. Research has, again and again, proven that recovery can be achieved even decades after stroke. The period after the wave of natural recovery is not the beginning of the end, only the end of the beginning. After the wave has lost its force, progress becomes slower and harder to achieve. Once the wave ends, most stroke survivors slow down or quit.

WHAT PRECAUTIONS SHOULD BE TAKEN?

After natural recovery has ended you will have the responsibility of steering your own recovery. After the period of natural recovery is when your real work begins.

✳　　✳　　✳

TIPS FOR THE CAREGIVER

If you've read this far, you know that the message of this book to the stroke survivor is simple: *The highest level of recovery is only possible with relentless hard work.* Caregivers have an equally simple reminder: *Your job is to help facilitate that hard work.*

From the shock of first learning that a loved one has had a stroke, and often for decades to come, caring for a stroke survivor can be overwhelming. The sprint of activity in the **acute** stage gives way to the full marathon of recovery. The stroke survivor has to do all of the work of recovering, but the caregiver provides support, resources, energy, and time. All of these elements are essential to the recovery effort.

Stroke is different from other forms of diseases of the nervous system. Most diseases of the nervous system are progressive (i.e., the symptoms get worse over time; e.g., Alzheimer's, Parkinson's, multiple sclerosis). Stroke is not progressive, and stroke survivors have the chance of recovering what the stroke took—with a lot of hard work. The possibility of recovery puts extra stress on caregivers because it is often difficult to know when to push forward and when to back off. Further stress is added when caregivers believe that the success or failure of the stroke survivor is dependent on their care, encouragement, and support.

HOW IS IT DONE?

Next to the stroke survivor, caregivers have the most to gain from the survivor's fullest possible recovery. Aiding in the recovery effort has the caregiver fighting on two fronts:

- Helping the stroke survivor recover
- Maintaining their own sanity

It's a tricky balance and, much like recovery from stroke itself, full of ups and downs. Here are some suggestions for the caregiver

- What caregivers should do for themselves:
  — Contact your rehabilitation doctor (**physiatrist**) and other rehabilitation personnel to educate you in the proper transfer techniques (e.g., from bed to standing or from chair to couch), fall recovery (once someone has fallen, when and how to help), tricks to facilitate activities of daily living, etc. A solid foundation in these basics will help the caregiver help the stroke survivor.
  — Keep records of progress made, and note any other pertinent information (lists of medications, important phone numbers, etc.).
  — Keep in mind that many caregivers believe that working with their stroke survivor is an enriching and fulfilling experience.
  — The recovery of a stroke survivor calls for the need of a coach, mentor, teacher, friend, and confidant. Having all these roles assumed by a spouse or any other single individual is a recipe for burnout. Caregivers who wear themselves down are less effective in helping to manage the recovery process. Friends, children, professional caregivers, therapists, and doctors can share in the effort.

- What caregivers should do for the stroke survivor:
  — Provide the infrastructure for the stroke survivor to succeed. This may involve anything from ordering exercise equipment to doing research.
  — Allow the stroke survivor to challenge him- or herself. For example, allow the stroke survivor the time to get the sentence out, rather than finishing the sentence for him, or time to cut his own food despite the difficulty.
- The caregiver can do three things, every day, that will help keep recovery on track.
  1. Be a cheerleader. Provide praise. Point out progress. Encourage. Allow mistakes, but also catch the survivor doing things right.
  2. Be a teacher. Help facilitate proper technique and quality of movement.
  3. Modify whatever skill is worked on to be challenging. There are many physical challenges that are part of life after stroke. These challenges are, ironically, the best tools for recovery from stroke. Many of these challenges can push the stroke survivor into uncomfortable but productive territory. Resisting the urge to make life easier for a stroke survivor helps lead to gains. There are single stroke survivors who claim that they have recovered because they *had* to recover. There was no one around to "do for them."

After a stroke, survivors are given a tough message. To someone who has not had a stroke it might sound a bit like this: "You now have to learn to play piano, learn gymnastics, and learn French. And you have to do it all at the same time. Oh yeah, and you've lost your job." Understanding the depth of the challenge of recovery will help the caregiver appreciate the spiritual turning point that recovery becomes.

WHAT PRECAUTIONS SHOULD BE TAKEN?

Caregivers who are stressed have a higher rate of depression, illness, and even death than caregivers who effectively deal with the stress and take care of themselves.

An essential resource is provided by the National Institutes of Health (NIH). It is a website that provides a portal to hundreds of pages of caregiver support, suggestions, and organizations. You can find it at:

www.nlm.nih.gov/medlineplus/caregivers.html

Safeguarding the Recovery Investment

STAY OFF THE KILLING FLOOR

Falls are a serious health threat to everyone, but falls are especially dangerous to stroke survivors. Here are some scary statistics:

- Up to 70% of patients have a fall in the 6 months after their stroke.
- Stroke survivors are two times as likely to fall, and three times as likely to be injured in a fall, than those who have not had a stroke.
- If anyone over 65 has a fall that results in a hospital stay, they have a 50% chance of dying in the next year.
- A stroke survivor is up to four times more likely to break her hip than people of the same age who have not had a stroke.
- Because of falls, medical costs each year in the United States are approximately $70 billion.

Stroke survivors are much more likely to fall than aged-matched folks who have not had a stroke. Stroke survivors tend to fall because:

- They experience weakness on the affected side of the body. Weakness can cause loss of balance. Weakness can increase the chances of a fall toward the paretic (or paralyzed) side.
- They have a loss of sensation on the affected side. Loss of sensation in stroke survivors takes any or all of following three forms:
  — Loss of feeling on the skin, like light touch and temperature
  — Numbness in the affected limbs
  — Loss of proprioception. Loss of proprioception makes it impossible for the stroke survivor to know what position his leg is in. That is, if a stroke survivor's eyes are closed, he cannot "feel" where the leg is.

Weakness and poor balance control on the affected side often cause the stroke survivor's weight to be thrown toward that "bad" side during a loss of balance. Once balance is lost, the stroke survivor tends to fall toward the weak side and is unable to brace for the fall with the paretic (weak) arm and hand. During the fall, there is a tendency toward hitting a particularly vulnerable part of the hip, the part that sticks out on the side of the leg, called the **greater trochanter**. This sort of fall can lead to a fracture (break) of the upper leg bone or any boney part of the hip joint.

Falls can not only cause hip fractures, but other broken bones in other parts of the body and/or other types of injuries.

For a variety of reasons stroke survivors who fall are likely to break their hip. Repairing a broken hip is major surgery. To repair a broken hip, either the femur (the bone that forms the top of the leg and forms part of the hip joint) is fastened together with screws and plates or the entire hip joint is replaced.

These sorts of surgeries are not without complications. You can develop:

- A pressure sore or blisters
- Lung infections
- Urinary infections
- Surgical complications (e.g., tissue infections)
- Orthopedic complications
- Gait deviations (limp)
- **Thrombosis** or **embolisms**, which are types of blood clots that can cause another stroke

And, to top it all off, if you break a hip you have a greater chance of having another hip fracture.

Falls can be devastating for stroke survivors. Falls can:

- Halt progress toward physical recovery
- Kill (either from the fall itself or from complications arising from the fall)
- Break any number of a wide variety of bones
- Forever end the ability to walk
- Increase the fear of walking
- Reduce the amount and quality of walking
- Lead to wheelchair confinement
- Forever make walking painful
- Lead to a hip replacement or surgery that reattaches the bone

Convalescence from a fall can lead to:

- Clot formation
- Bed sores
- Loss of strength both of muscles and bones, even those not injured in the fall
- Reduced cardiovascular stamina

And physical injury is not the only damaging result of a fall. Once someone has had an incident, the fear of falling again often causes people to restrict cherished activities like shopping, eating out, and attending church. Because of reduced involvement in the community, falls can result in social isolation and depression. Falls also make stroke survivors fearful to work on recovery, especially recovery efforts that involve standing, stair climbing, or walking.

HOW IS IT DONE?

Here are some suggestions for reducing falls:

- Exercise regularly. Strong muscles help reduce falls.
- Wear sturdy shoes outside and inside. Do not walk in slippers, flip-flops, walk barefoot, or in socks.
- Overall, allow for more lighting in your home.
- Clear away all items that you can trip over. Make sure pets are kept out of the walking area.
- Do not use throw rugs that can slide or move.
- Place often used items within easy reach to eliminate the need for a step stool.
- Make sure there are handrails on stairs.
- Have your doctor review your medications regarding their potential influence on falling. There is a direct relationship between the number of medications taken (no matter what kind) and the risk of falling.
- There are tests that can be done in the clinic to predict if you are at risk for falls. These tests include:
  — Five-Times-Sit-to-Stand Test
  — Timed Up and Go
  — Functional Reach Test
  — Berg Balance Scale
  — Falls Efficacy Scale

These tests are usually done by physical or occupational therapists.

- Have vision checked yearly.
- Have a physical or occupational therapist visit your home to make sure your home is fall proof.
- Consider protective padding. There are discrete hip pads that can be worn inside undergarments to protect hips during a fall. There are many manufacturers producing hip pads of this sort.
- The bathroom is a uniquely hazardous room. Many hard surfaces within a small area combined with wet and slippery floors make bathrooms potentially dangerous. The need to transfer from bath/shower and toilet make bathrooms a challenge to fall proof.

Here are suggestions for keeping your bathroom safe:
— Install grab-bars in the tub and shower.
— Install grab-bars next to the toilet.
— Place non-slip mats in bathtub and shower.
— Make tile nonslip, with chemical treatments that etch the surface.
— Have adequate lighting on the path to and in bathroom so that it's easy to see during nighttime trips.
— Don't lock the bathroom door, in case you need help.

WHAT PRECAUTIONS SHOULD BE TAKEN?

The main precaution is *do not ignore this chapter*. This may be the most important chapter in this book. Falls kill. When told of these facts, many people think that clinicians are just trying to scare them. In this case it is a healthy fear. Take precautions.

✳   ✳   ✳

REDUCE THE RISK OF ANOTHER STROKE

Many stroke survivors and their caregivers do not know the complete list of possible stroke symptoms. If you've already had a stroke, you have a 35% chance of having another one. It is essential that you know all the symptoms of stroke, not just the symptoms that were experienced during your previous stroke.

HOW IS IT DONE?

Learn the symptoms of stroke. The easiest way is to start at the top of the head and move downward.

- Skull: sudden, severe headache and/or dizziness, with no known cause
- Eyes: sudden trouble seeing in one or both eyes
- Ears: sudden trouble understanding
- Face: facial weakness

- Mouth: sudden trouble speaking
- Body: sudden numbness, weakness, or paralysis on one side of the body

There is a quick, easy, and effective way of determining if someone is having a stroke. Developed by researchers at the University of Cincinnati, the *Cincinnati Prehospital Stroke Scale* helps people recognize a stroke by asking the individual to do three things:

1. Ask the individual to smile.
   - Are both sides of the face equal? Is one side of the face drooping?
2. Ask the person to speak a simple sentence clearly such as: "The sky is blue in Cincinnati."
   - Listen carefully to the quality of speech. Are words being slurred?
3. Ask him or her to raise both arms.
   - Does one arm drift? Are both arms held at the same height?

If the individual has difficulty with any of these tasks call 9-1-1 immediately, and describe the symptoms to the dispatcher.

React quickly! Some of the newer medications for reducing the impact of a stroke have to be administered within the first 2 or 3 hours after stroke, so recognizing stroke *quickly* is essential to surviving and recovering from a stroke. A stroke is the process of brain cells dying. Every *minute* of a stroke destroys almost 2 million nerve cells in the brain. Time saved is brain saved.

WHAT PRECAUTIONS SHOULD BE TAKEN?

Know the symptoms of stroke. Remember: From the top down—Skull, Eyes, Ears, Face, Mouth, and Body.

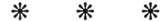

PROTECT YOUR BONES

Stroke survivors are at a much higher risk for breaking bones than the general population. Stroke survivors have up to four times the risk for breaking bones. There are two main reasons for this:

- People who have had a stroke have a tendency toward high blood levels of an amino acid, homocysteine. Homocysteine can weaken bones.
- The lack of weight-bearing activities such as walking and other load-bearing activities puts less pressure on bones. The decrease in pressure may reduce the thickness of bones, leading to osteoporosis (**Wolf's law**).

It is essential that you have a plan for maintaining bone health and bone strength. This plan might include any or all of the following:

- Diagnostic tests (bone density tests can be done by your doctor to determine if bones are at risk for fracture)
- Assessment of risk for falls
- Addition of bone-building medications or supplements
- Performance of any of a variety of forms of physical activity, including resistive exercises and a daily routine of walking

HOW IS IT DONE?

There are many techniques to increase bone strength and reduce the risk of damage to bones, such as the following:

- As discussed in (see Weight Up, page 107) resistance training (and or weight training) will build bone thickness (**Wolf's law**).
- Fall prevention steps will decrease fractures (see Stay Off the Killing Floor, page 48).
- Walking, as part of a daily routine, can reduce bone loss after stroke.
- A variety of medications can decrease or prevent bone loss and have the possibility of increasing bone strength. Ask your doctor about these medications.
- There are nutritional steps that can be taken to help bone health. Nutritional steps include supplementation with calcium, folic acid, and vitamin B12 and adequate protein intake, all of which can potentially build bone strength. There is some scientific evidence that vitamin K and D reduces osteoporosis in stroke survivors. Sunlight may help build bones as well.
- There are many techniques that physical therapists can provide, which can improve balance and reduce falls. Have a physical therapist develop a balance training exercise program that you can do

safely at home. This should be part of your comprehensive home exercise program (see Get a Home Exercise Program, page 100).

WHAT PRECAUTIONS SHOULD BE TAKEN?

All of the steps you take to reduce fractures should be discussed with your doctor. Supplementation with vitamins, minerals, amino acids, and so forth may interfere with medications, so talk to your doctor before taking vitamin, mineral, amino acid, or herbal supplements.

✳   ✳   ✳

STRETCH OUT

Some stroke survivors have difficulty straightening their affected elbow because of muscle tightness (spasticity). The elbow is constantly bent, and it continues to stay bent, all day, every day. After a while, the structures around the elbow joint including muscles, skin, nerves, blood vessels, and other **soft tissue** shorten. Once this tissue shortens, the tissue will remain shortened forever. Straightening the elbow becomes impossible. The elbow can't even be straightened with the help of the unaffected hand, or with the help of someone else. This inability to straighten a joint is called **contracture**. Contracture eliminates any possibility of the joint recovering its original arc of movement. Once there is contracture, surgery to lengthen the shortened soft tissue is necessary. This is a serious condition with serious consequences.

As stroke survivors progress beyond being flaccid (limp), muscles tend to become **spastic** (tight). This tightness can lead to contracture. Safely and effectively stretching the muscles on the affected side should be done constantly and faithfully so contracture does not develop. Constant stretching of muscles will help retain the full length of those muscles (and other soft tissue) and retain the greatest possible range of motion. Stretching will conserve soft tissue length and protect joint **range of motion**, both of which are essential to any further recovery. If the best possible treatment for you becomes available, contracture will eliminate any possible benefit. If soft tissue length is maintained, it will provide the perfect template for recovery techniques as they become available. Other reasons that stretching is so important:

1. Stretching may provide a short-term reduction in spasticity. It is common for therapists and other clinicians to believe that stretching reduces spasticity. But because spasticity is a brain problem and not a muscle problem, copious stretching will not reduce spasticity permanently. However, there is some research showing that stretching provides some short-term reduction in spasticity.

2. Stretching reduces the soreness sometimes associated with recovery efforts. Much of recovery from stroke involves repetitive practice, which can work muscles in ways they are not used to. This can lead to something called delayed-onset muscle soreness or DOMS. This phenomenon usually develops one to several days after the actual practice. Stretching can reduce or eliminate DOMS.

3. Stretching is good for you. Stretching is of benefit to muscle and other soft tissue, whether affected by the stroke or not. Retaining flexibility keeps your body young. Stretching will benefit muscles on the unaffected side, the trunk, and in other areas of the body.

4. Stretching makes every movement easier. Muscle uses spasticity to protect itself from being torn. After stroke, muscles sense that something is severely wrong and send out panic signals to the spinal cord. The spinal cord tells the muscles to protect themselves by tightening. This process causes spasticity (see page 138 for a full description of spasticity). Both the flexors (muscles that "close" a joint) and extensors (muscles that "open" a joint) may have spasticity after stroke, but the muscles that flex joints tend to be bigger and more powerful than the muscles that extend joints. For example, after stroke the affected arm and hand tends to posture so that all the joints are flexed.

   - The typical posture of the **hemiparetic** stroke survivor is with the arm across the front of the body with the elbow, wrist, and fingers bent. This posture is simply the flexor muscles "beating" the extensor muscles every time. There is relatively more spastic pull on the muscles that bend joints than straighten joints.

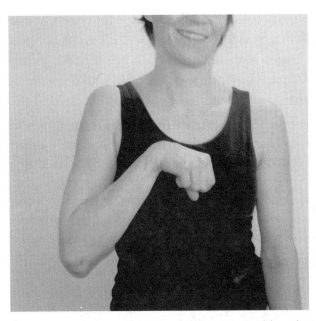

This posture is a defense mechanism for the arm and hand. Consider the alternative. If the arm were limp, it would flail by your side in constant danger of tearing muscle, damaging joints, and bumping into nearby objects. Basic protection comes from the fact that all the flexor muscles pull the arm and hand near the body.

The same is true in the leg and foot. The calf muscles are big and bulky and are actually comprised of two muscles that lift the entire weight of the body while walking. This muscle points the foot downward at the ankle. The muscle, in a "spastic war" with the huge calf muscles, is a much smaller muscle, which only has to lift the foot. If both muscles are in a spastic battle, guess which muscle wins? The "winning" muscle loses by remaining in a shortened position. Over time the muscles left in a shortened position shorten permanently. This is one of the reasons lifting the foot after stroke is so hard and why **ankle-foot orthoses** (**AFO**) are often prescribed.

HOW IS IT DONE?

Range of motion (ROM) refers to the complete arc of available, non-painful movement of a joint. For example, at the elbow, the ROM would be from the elbow fully bent to the elbow fully straight. To prevent contractures, perform range-of-motion exercises on yourself, or have a trained caregiver perform these exercises. The joint should be brought through its complete *nonpainful* range of motion several times a day. Many times these range-of-motion exercises are something that stroke survivors can do for themselves.

The best advice available for stretching will come from a plan set up by your OT and PT. Typically, an occupational therapist would develop a stretching program for the arm and hand, and a physical therapist would do the same for the leg and foot. Ask therapists for specific stretches that, while remaining safe, are as aggressive as possible, and can be done at home. See the precaution section prior to attempting any stretching. Here are some general suggestions for stretching the muscles that are most at risk for contracture. Focus stretching on the following muscle groups (it is never a single muscle but a group that works together, which need stretching).

Muscles that most need stretching in the arm and hand include:

- The finger flexors (the muscles that make a fist)
- The wrist flexors (the muscles that bend the wrist in toward the arm)
- The elbow flexors (the muscles that bend the elbow)
- The shoulder adductors (the muscles that bring the upper arm close to the body)
- The shoulder internal rotators (the muscles that bring the forearm across the front of the trunk)

Muscles that most need stretching in the leg and foot include:

- The hip adductors (the muscles that bring one leg toward the other at the hip)
- The hip flexors (the muscles that bend the hip toward the chest)
- The knee flexors (the muscles that bend the knee)
- The ankle plantar flexors (the muscles that push the foot down. In standing this would be a "heel-up" position)
- Toe flexors (the muscles that bend the toes down)

Remember, these are the muscles that need to be stretched, so the stretch would go in the direction opposite of the movement described previously. For example, if you want to stretch the elbow flexors that bend the elbow, then you would stretch by moving the elbow in the opposite direction, which would involve straightening the elbow. See the precautions portion of this section before any stretching program is started.

A note about stretching the wrist and fingers: If the fingers are stretched without also extending the wrist, then only some of the muscles will get stretched. This is because the same muscles that cross the wrist also cross all the joints in the fingers. Effective stretching involves extending the wrist at the same time as the fingers are stretched (prayer position). Conversely, if the wrist is being stretched, then the fingers have to be extended. The fingers and wrist have to be stretched at the same time because the same muscles cross both the finger and wrist joints.

This is just one of many examples of how stretching may have a bit more complexity than you might imagine. Therapists are experts at taking the guesswork out of stretching. If a high-quality stretching program is developed, it will be effective for the rest of your life. Therapists will be able to develop a stretching program for you in one to three sessions.

Stroke survivors often ask, "How often should I stretch?" Ideally you would stretch the affected side muscles as much as the unaffected muscles are naturally stretched. Consider the muscles that bend the elbow. How many times a day is your unaffected "good" elbow straightened? This gives us a window on what muscles require to stay healthy. Providing the same amount of stretching as the unaffected side may not be feasible due to time constraints. Still, we can assume that an effective self-stretching program needs much more effort than is usually given.

Another effective treatment to encourage the lengthening of muscles on their way to contracture is a long, slow stretch over an extended period of time. In a process called "serial casting," the joint is casted in a lengthened position, which helps the muscle permanently lengthen. Serial casting is usually done by specially trained physical or occupational therapists. Serial casting is done for cases where spasticity is very high and regular stretching programs are ineffective.

WHAT PRECAUTIONS SHOULD BE TAKEN?

Sometimes spasticity is so strong that stretching a group of muscles is impossible because of the tightness of the muscle. This will result in certain contracture. If you are unable to take any joint through its range of motion, even with the help of your unaffected side or with help of a caregiver, consult either a physiatrist or neurologist. There are a variety of medications that might decrease the spasticity that is leading you toward contracture. It used to be that the only spasticity medications available were taken orally. Oral spasticity medications often leave patients tired because these medications are muscle relaxants, which affect all the muscles of the body, not just the spastic ones. New developments in the delivery of spasticity medication now allow doctors to target only the muscle groups that are spastic (see Give Spasticity the One-Two Punch, page 145).

When stretching muscles, carefully follow the instructions of the healthcare professional who has taught the stretches. Pain always means, "Stop the stretch!" Even something as simple as **passive range of motion** (having the joint moved without the power of the muscles surrounding the joint), whether done on yourself, or done on some else, can be dangerous. Muscles, ligaments, and joints can be torn and veins, arteries, and nerves can be damaged. On the other hand, once your therapists and your doctor develop a safe stretching program, the biggest precaution is not stretching enough!

✻   ✻   ✻

SHOULDER CARE 101

Many stroke survivors have shoulder pain. The shoulder joint is at risk for trauma, dislocation, and pain because the shoulder joint is designed for movement, not strength. After stroke the muscles that normally keep the shoulder stable are often too weak to hold the joint in place. Because of this, the shoulder is vulnerable to dislocation (called subluxation). Subluxation can lead to painful and limited movement.

Even if no dislocation has occurred, the shoulder can be a problem after stroke. Many of the problems that the shoulder has after stroke are caused by the reduction in overall shoulder movement. The typical way the arm is held after stroke is across, and close to, the chest. The shoulder joint is usually held like this because of:

- Limited strength of the muscles that move the arm away from the body
- Spasticity that makes the joint difficult to move

• Stiffness and pain that limits movement

All these elements lead to the shoulder no longer being moved through its normal **active** and **passive range of motion**. The lack of normal movement in the shoulder joint causes the soft tissue (muscle, nerves, blood vessels, etc.) around the joint to shorten. This can make movement uncomfortable, painful, and difficult. In some cases, the soft tissue shortens so much that movement is impossible. This is called **contracture**. The loss of normal shoulder movement and other negative aspects brought to bear on the shoulder by stroke (e.g., reduced blood flow, muscle atrophy, etc.) can magnify shoulder pain after stroke. Also, the shoulder joint can be at risk because people will attempt to help you move by grabbing your affected arm, which can injure the shoulder joint.

Probably the worst stressor on the shoulder joint can be delivered with pulleys. Pulleys are handles attached to ropes. The ropes are attached to a wheel so that if you pull downward on one handle, the other handle (with the other arm and hand holding it) goes upward. Pulleys are available in most rehabilitation gyms. Therapists often use them to help patients with different disorders (not just stroke) "range" themselves (self-stretch). Pulleys can be dangerous for the weak-side shoulder of stroke survivors. Unless a doctor specifically suggests pulleys, decline their use. Other forms of aggressive "ranging" (putting the joint through, and beyond, its range of motion) with the aid of your "good" side, or with the aid of another person or machine should be considered cautiously. Aggressive ranging of the shoulder joint can damage the joint. Keep in mind, however, that proper, nonpainful stretching of the shoulder joint is necessary after stroke. The shoulder should be part of a comprehensive stretching program that takes all the joints on the affected side through their full, safe, and nonpainful passive range of motion.

HOW IS IT DONE?

It is important to focus attention on the affected shoulder to prevent injury, increase coordination, and keep muscles strong. This attention will allow for the largest possible potential toward recovery. Here are strategies that can help to protect the shoulder:

- Physiotaping (also known as simply as taping or strapping) is a way of taping the shoulder to protect the joint and allow for correct movement.
- Positioning techniques are simply defined as the way the shoulder is left to rest in order to protect the joint.
- Particular types of shoulder slings can protect the shoulder.
- The best way to protect the shoulder joint is to strengthen the muscles around the joint and adequately and gently stretch the joint. Occupational therapists are experts in exercises that aid the shoulder joint. Exercises that build muscle to support the shoulder are essential. Rehabilitation specialists can provide exercises that lie within the ability of the stroke survivor. Consult your doctor and rehabilitation health-care worker and ask them to provide a plan to allow for the greatest possible potential toward shoulder recovery.
- Many researchers believe that the best thing you can do for your shoulder is to increase movement in the hand. The shoulder will develop strength and coordination naturally if it is used to aid the hand in getting to where it needs to be in real-world ways. The work of getting the hand functional can have a significant effect on the muscles that control the shoulder. Some therapists and researchers believe that a useable hand will actually resolve dislocation of the shoulder. As the hand is used more, the shoulder muscles are used more. As the shoulder muscles are used, they strengthen, which pulls the shoulder joint together. Ideas to get the hand "back in the game" are discussed in Get Your Hand Back, page 74.

WHAT PRECAUTIONS SHOULD BE TAKEN?

Consult your doctor regarding any pain that affects function of the shoulder. Don't make the mistake of not consulting a doctor for pain that limits movement because reduced movement can lead to a downward spiral, causing shortening of the soft tissue that surrounds the joint, which leads to less movement and, in turn, can lead to more shortening of soft tissue. Periodically consult your occupational or physical therapist for proper exercises and other treatments and modalities to help support the weak-side shoulder.

❋　❋　❋

FIVE TESTS YOU SHOULD DO

Cardiovascular issues: You will often hear about how important they are to your overall health. For stroke survivors the impact of damaged and clogged arteries has already been felt. You might think that having a stroke is an isolated incident. But the truth is that stroke survivors have their stroke to thank for alerting them that all is not well with their blood vessels. Vascular disease is not isolated; it is a disease that usually shows up in the walls of many arteries at once. Arteries are the blood vessels, the plumbing if you will, that takes blood from your heart and delivers it to every one of the trillions of cells in your body. Arterial disease can happen in any number of vessels, and the fact that some arteries are diseased may not make much difference in your life. But in some organs, like the heart and brain, this disease process can kill you. Stroke survivors know what can happen in the brain when an artery clogs or bursts: Stroke. Most people know the impact of this disease in the heart, too: a heart attack. Arterial disease is 80% preventable. There are a few basic steps that you can take to keep your arteries healthy:

- Stop smoking
- Up with the good (HDL) and down with the bad (LDL) cholesterol
- Control diabetes
- Watch your weight
- Exercise

All of these efforts will benefit the health of your arteries. Once you put these efforts into practice, follow up by doing some simple tests. These tests will help you determine if your efforts are successful.

HOW IS IT DONE?

A series of tests that can reveal arterial health follows. Two of them, pulse rate and blood pressure (BP), should be done during the entire recovery process and, when feasible, during each recovery workout or session. Pulse and BP readings will provide essential information that will keep you safe as you continue to recover. Pulse rate and BP can also provide information about overall, long-term cardiovascular health and strength. Generally, the lower the numbers for both pulse and BP, the better. Your doctor can provide specific guidelines. Pulse and blood pressure should also be taken during periods of rest, as well, because resting pulse and resting blood pressure are key indicators of cardiovascular health (again, generally, the lower the better). Keep an ongoing record of these two measures. Your self-testing results will provide valuable information for your doctor and therapists, so bring the information with you when visiting health professionals. Knowing, by *heart*, your pulse and BP will help you know if you are remaining safe.

Here are a few basic tests that stroke survivors can do to keep track of the health of their arteries:

- *Take your blood pressure.* Digital blood pressure machines are inexpensive and easy to use. Bring your machine into your doctor's office to judge the machine's accuracy. Compare the doctor's reading against what your machine says. Your doctor will tell you what normal blood pressure is for you; normal varies from person to person depending on a number of factors, including the effects of certain medications.
- *Take your pulse.* (Many digital blood-pressure monitors take pulse as well.)

  Here is how to take pulse: look at a clock with a second hand. Place the tips of your "good-side" index and long fingers on the

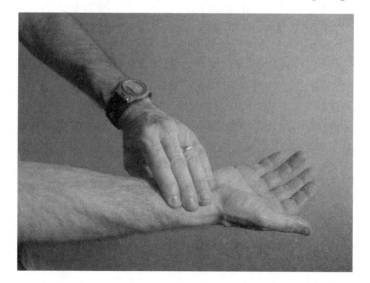

palm side of your other wrist, below the base of the thumb. Press lightly with your fingers, feeling the pulsing with your fingertips. Count the number of beats for 15 seconds. Multiply the number of beats by four. That will be your pulse per minute.

Ask your doctor what the parameters should be. Be aware of what your resting pulse should be and of the highest pulse you can safely maintain during exercise. Much of what is suggested in this book is aerobic exercise (exercise involving the heart and lungs) and aerobic exercise increases heart (pulse) rate. So knowing the safe range of pulse rate is important for safety.

- *Have cholesterol checked by a doctor.* It is a blood test. There are at-home blood tests, but their accuracy may be questionable.
- *Monitor blood sugar.* You can do this even if you are not diabetic but suspect something may be wrong with your blood sugar. There are inexpensive, over-the-counter blood-sugar tests at your drugstore.
- *Take your **waist-to-hip ratio**.* Waist-to-hip ratio is the best predictor of cardiovascular death. **Central obesity** (carrying fat around the middle or apple-shape, where the waist is larger than the hips) increases the risk of stroke, heart disease, high blood pressure, and diabetes. Carrying fat in the hips and thighs, or having a pear shape, is not as harmful to your health. You can calculate your waist to hip ratio by dividing your waist measurement by your hip measurement.

Waist: Relaxed, measured around at belly button.

Hips: Measure around the widest part of the hip-bones.

For instance:

Measurement at the waist = 34

Measurement at the hips = 37

$34 \div 37 = 0.92$

Ratios above 0.80 for women and 0.95 for men increases the risk of stroke, heart disease, high blood pressure, and diabetes.

WHAT PRECAUTIONS SHOULD BE TAKEN?

Home tests are great. They are convenient, and they tell you what you need to know. But these tests are done most accurately when skilled health-care professionals do them. Lack of accuracy of machines, as well as poor collection techniques can provide false readings.

If you suspect that a reading (pulse rate, blood pressure, etc.) is cause for concern, contact your doctor or call emergency services (911).

Cool Treatment Options

CONSTRAINT-INDUCED THERAPY FOR THE ARM AND HAND

The basis of all recovery from stroke is **neuroplasticity** (see Use Your Fantastic Plastic Brain, page 6). There are several ways of activating the neuroplastic process. The most famous is **constraint-induced therapy** (**CIT**). In traditional CIT therapy, the unaffected hand and arm is immobilized with either a sling and/or mitt while the affected hand and arm does a lot of **repetitive practice**. The exercises are repeated for 6 to 8 hours a day, for 2 to 3 weeks. If this schedule seems tough, consider the fact that athletes and musicians often spend multiple hours a day for months doing specific exercises. And they do it year in and year out. A stroke survivor who is trying to recover is just like an athlete or musician; she is always trying to rewire her brain by practicing with her limbs.

HOW IS IT DONE?

There are facilities that provide structured CIT programs. The most famous is the Taub Therapy Clinic, located in Birmingham, Alabama. This clinic is run by Edward Taub, PhD, originator of CIT. This clinical intervention is intense; it lasts for either 2 or 3 weeks, and it is done multiple hours a day.

- Taub Therapy Clinic, Birmingham, AL
  Website: www.taubtherapy.com
  Phone: 866-554-TAUB

This therapy is expensive because it requires many hours of occupational and physical therapy, and a therapist's time is expensive.

Another form of CIT is called *modified* constraint-induced therapy (mCIT). Developed by stroke-recovery researcher Dr. Stephen J. Page, mCIT is now available in many facilities across the United States. Modified constraint-induced therapy is different from traditional CIT in terms of the number of hours a day that are needed to see the treating therapist. With classic mCIT, the stroke survivor sees the therapist three times a week, but wears a restraint on the affected arm and hand for up to 5 hours a day during active hours when he or she is at home. Therapists have been modifying mCIT ever since the mid 1990s to fit their set of skills and incorporate the resources of their particular hospital or rehab facility.

Here is a partial list of facilities that provide some form of CIT or mCIT:

- Kessler Institute for Rehabilitation, West Orange, NJ
  Website: www.kessler-rehab.com
  Phone: 973-731-3600

- Burke Rehabilitation Hospital, White Plains, NY
  Website: www.burke.org
  Phone: 914-597-2326

- Garden State Physical Therapy, Hasbrouck Heights, NJ
  Website: www.GardenStatePT.com
  Phone: 201-288-4884

- Sunnyview Rehabilitation Hospital, Schenectady, NY
  Website: www.sunnyview.org
  Phone: 518-382-4569

- Magee Rehabilitation Hospital, Philadelphia, PA
  Website: www.mageerehab.org
  Phone: 800-966-2433

- Braintree Rehabilitation Hospital, Braintree, MA
  Website: www.braintreerehabhospital.com
  Phone: 781-348-2500

- Fairlawn Rehabilitation Hospital, Worcester, MA
  Website: www.fairlawnrehab.org
  Phone: 508-471-9322

- CarePartners Health Services, Asheville, NC
  Website: www.carepartners.org/outpatient.html
  Phone: 828-277-4800

- Emory Healthcare's HealthConnections, Atlanta, GA
  Website: www.emoryhealthcare.org
  Phone: 404-778-7777

- Siskin Hospital for Physical Rehabilitation, Chattanooga, TN
  Website: www.siskinrehab.org/patient/costraint.asp
  Phone: 423-634-1389

- Rehabilitation Institute of Chicago, Chicago, IL
  Website: www.ric.org
  Phone: 866-999-3344

- University of Michigan Health System, MedRehab, Ann Arbor, MI
  Website: www.med.umich.edu
  Phone: 734-998-7911

- Advanced Recovery Rehab Center, Sherman Oaks, CA
  Website: www.advancedrecovery.org
  Phone: 818-386-1231

Constraint-induced therapy (and mCIT) will not work if there is no jumping-off point. Research shows that you need some movement in the hand to start with. Here are some of the tests that researchers and clinicians have used to determine if CIT or mCIT is appropriate for someone:

- The ability to actively lift hand, thumb, and at least two fingers from a relaxed position
- The ability to release a grasped tennis ball
- The ability to pick up and release a rag off a tabletop using any type of grasp/release

Researchers have also used even lower standards. One such standard is simply the ability to wipe a towel across a table. Therapists have used similar standards in the clinic.

Can someone do CIT alone at home? Certainly, there are elements of CIT that you can do at home, safely, and with little training and setup. But there are also mistakes that can be made during CIT. Mistakes can make the therapy ineffective and worse, can put the stroke survivor at risk of injury. CIT should be done, at least to begin with, while working with an occupational or physical therapist. Constraint-induced therapy is simply a way to stop, and reverse, what researchers call **learned nonuse**. Learned nonuse is when stroke survivors essentially teach themselves not to use their affected limbs. Here's how it works.

You try to use the affected side and you find movement difficult. Then you try to use the "good" side and everything is much easier. This causes you to do more with the "good" limb and less with the "bad" limb. The less the "bad" limb moves, the more the movement becomes difficult. As a result, you use the limb even less, which means even less dedicated brainpower,

LEARNED NONUSE

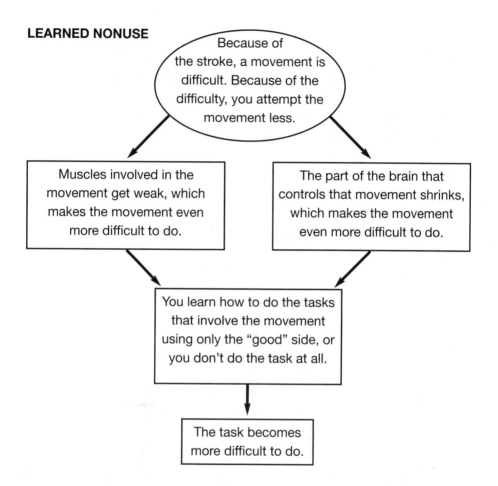

Because of the stroke, a movement is difficult. Because of the difficulty, you attempt the movement less.

Muscles involved in the movement get weak, which makes the movement even more difficult to do.

The part of the brain that controls that movement shrinks, which makes the movement even more difficult to do.

You learn how to do the tasks that involve the movement using only the "good" side, or you don't do the task at all.

The task becomes more difficult to do.

and so the downward spiral continues. In this way the stroke survivor "learns" not to use the affected limb. Researchers know from the concept of **neuroplasticity** that the more you do a movement, the more brainpower is devoted to that movement. The opposite is also true: as you use the limb less, less brainpower is directed to that movement. The less brainpower dedicated to the movement, the worse the limb moves. Constraint-induced therapy attempts to reverse the downward spiral of learned nonuse by forcing you to use the "bad" limb. Constraint-induced therapy uses **repetitive practice** of the affected limb to promote recovery. The small parts, called "component parts" of an entire task are practiced over and over. As each of the component parts of the task are learned, all the parts are put together and the entire task is practiced. The process of developing component parts needed for one task helps with other tasks as well. Consider that component part of lifting your arm at the shoulder as part of reaching for a cup. Once the ability to lift the arm is learned, it can be used to do many other tasks from writing (to get the arm to the table) to turning on a light switch. This process of building small parts of a movement into an effective whole movement is the basis of CIT.

Constraint-induced therapy should be done with a trained rehabilitation professional. Once you understand the basic ideas behind using CIT to recover movement, you can easily use the spirit of CIT and mCIT in other areas of your recovery.

REVERSING LEARNED NONUSE

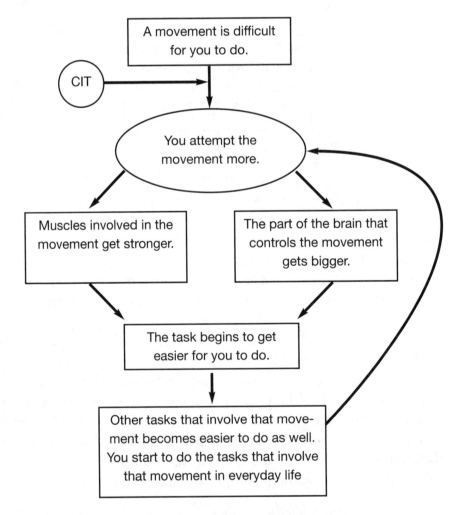

Leg constraint-induced therapy (leg CIT)

The spirit of CIT is that the unaffected limb essentially *does nothing*, while the affected limb does all the work. Research into leg CIT lags far behind arm/hand CIT because it is difficult to respect the spirit of CIT *and* keep you safe. Remember, CIT involves constraining, with a sling and/or mitt, the "good" arm and hand. A quick look at leg CIT reveals the problem. How do you safely constrain a leg? How do you have only one limb do all the work and still engage in the primary function of the legs— walking? Leg CIT has another problem. The core of CIT involves practice with the "bad" side for several hours (5-8) a day. You can survive this tough schedule when doing arm CIT because you are sitting most of the time, and the muscles of the arm are small, relative to the leg. Since the leg muscles are much bigger than the arm muscles, you burn much more energy. This makes the harsh scheduling of CIT difficult to maintain.

Because of these inherent problems, leg CIT is rarely done clinically. Clinics that attempt this treatment use similar techniques to those used in arm/hand CIT. Leg CIT involves a lot of intense exercises for the affected leg. The goals of these exercises are twofold. First, the idea is to strengthen the muscles of the "bad" leg so that the limb is at least as strong as the unaffected leg. Second, this strategy provides many repetitions of component parts of walking (i.e., **dorsiflexion** or lifting the foot) to cause the necessary **neuroplastic** change.

WHAT PRECAUTIONS SHOULD BE TAKEN?

Make sure, before any CIT or mCIT program is started, that the version that the facility or therapist is using is shown to be effective in research that is published in **peer-reviewed** literature.

DO NOT constrain the unaffected hand and arm unless under the supervision of an MD or therapist. There are safety issues that must be considered when restricting the unaffected extremity. Constraining the unaffected arm and hand can lead to falls, burns, and other dangers.

Lower-extremity CIT exists but has to be done under the direct supervision of a therapist. Some of the facilities that offer CIT for the arm and hand also have CIT programs for the leg. Never attempt lower-extremity CIT without therapist supervision. DO NOT tie up the leg and or foot.

Constraint of the lower extremity is not done in any form of lower-extremity CIT.

* * *

GET YOUR HAND BACK

Generally speaking, the shoulder, elbow, and wrist are simply delivery systems for the hand. That is, the entire arm exists to bring the hand to where it needs to be. If the hand can be used in some sort of real-world way, all the muscles of the arm will work very hard to transport the hand. This hard work will help the entire arm recover.

But what if your hand does not yet work? Typically the hand is the last body part to recover. Arm recovery tends to begin in muscles and joints close to the body and move down the limb, toward the hand. Stroke survivors typically regain movement in this order:

> 1st—The muscles that move the shoulder blade
> 2nd—The muscles that move the shoulder joint (which moves the upper arm)
> 3rd—The muscles that move the elbow
> 4th—The muscles that rotate the forearm (palm up and palm down)
> 5th—The muscles that move the wrist
> 6th—The muscles that move the hand and fingers

Remember, the arm has a strong chance of recovering if the hand is working. But, because the hand comes back last, it is impossible to use the hand to help recovery in the rest of the arm. Recently however, researchers, entrepreneurs, and bioengineers have begun to solve the riddle of the hand. What has come of this research and experimentation has been the clinical use of a variety of gizmos, orthotics, machines, and techniques to "jump start" the hand.

HOW IS IT DONE?

How to jump start the hand depends on how much movement the hand has to begin with. Stroke survivors often grossly underestimate the movement in their hands. They tend to think that since the hand is not useful in any real-world way that any movement it has is not important. But a small amount of movement is important to one thing: recovery.

If you have any movement, in any joint, you can build on that movement by using **repetitive practice**. Repetitive practice means using the little movement you have to, over and over, try to "hit the end ranges" of that movement. In the fingers, this would mean opening and closing the fingers as much as possible. "Hitting the end ranges" would involve extra focus on the tail end of both of those movements. So you would open the fingers as much as possible and then try to open them just a little bit further. Then you would try to close the hand and then close it a little bit more.

The movement to open the hand may not amount to much more than the ability to relax the fingers enough to allow the fingers to "relax open." This ability to relax the fingers so they open slightly is important because it takes two to tango. The muscle that has to open the fingers has to fire, but equally important, the muscles that close the fingers have to relax. It is this dance between the muscles that presents the challenge, when you try, in whatever small way that you can, to open and then close your hand. Once you can open and close even one finger, repeat it for as long as you can tolerate it. Do it while you watch TV, talk on the phone, wherever and whenever. The other fingers and, eventually, the thumb, will follow if you try to repeat, over and over, the grasp-release movement of opening and closing the fingers.

But what if you have *no* movement? Or what if, as is the case with most stroke survivors, you can make a tight fist, but releasing that fist is impossible? This is where the machines and gizmos can help.

- One sort of machine that you can try uses cyclic electrical stimulation. This is simply electrical stimulation to the muscles that open the hand. These muscles are located on the back of the forearm. The machine simply stimulates the hand to open, and then the machine stops the stimulation. On and off it goes usually for 5 seconds or so of hand opening, followed by 10 seconds or so of no stimulation. These machines are relatively inexpensive, and once a doctor or therapist trains you on the machine, you can do it at home. If help is also needed to close the hand then the machine can be programmed to first open, then provide no stimulation, and then close the hand.

- *EMG-based electrical stimulation.* These machines ask for some sort of effort before the electrical stimulation is sent into the muscles. There is either a sound or a visual cue to open the hand. Once the muscles fire, stimulation opens the hand. These machines are sensitive, so they can pick up muscle activity even if you can't see movement in the hand. These machines include the Mentamove, Biomove, and NeuroMove™.
- *Electrical stimulation orthotic.* This orthotic is rigid plastic that forms perfectly around the forearm and provides the stimulation to the muscles that need it. This orthotic has an advantage over other forms of electrical stimulation; you can move the arm and hand around and do real-world activities. The only orthotic to provide this is the Bioness H200™.
- *Spring-loaded finger extension orthotic.* This orthotic uses springs and pulleys attached to a rigid orthotic to facilitate opening the fingers. You can move the arm and hand around and do real-world activities while you perform grasping activities. The orthotic helps the fingers "release" once objects are grasped. The only orthotic to provide this is the SaeboFlex®.

Some of the machines suggested require specially trained therapists. In some cases, contacting the manufacturer is the best way to find where, in your area, therapists are using these machines. See Recovery Machines (page 169) for more information on all of the machines reviewed here.

All the machines have the potential of providing a small amount of voluntary movement. Once there is voluntary movement you can start doing repetitive practice on your own.

Here are two other ideas to help develop movement in the hand that do not involve machines.

- *Passively moving the joints.* Recent research has revealed that passively moving a joint will begin to slightly rewire the brain. This may provide a small spark to begin the neuroplastic process. Much more neuroplastic change will happen when you initiate the movement yourself, but for low-level stroke survivors, passively moving the joint may help. It is interesting to note that many of the robots used for rehabilitation, including the products made by Myomo™

(www.myomo.com), use *some* passive movement to promote recovery. These robots only help where help is needed, however. The more movement that you can do yourself, the more recovery you will get.

- *Repetitive practice into flexion.* Although it may not seem to make sense at first glace, tightening your fingers into a fist may help to gain control over your hand. The reason that stroke survivors have a hard time opening the hand is spasticity in the muscles that close the hand and fingers. As discussed in "Neuroplastic Beats Spastic," spasticity is caused by too much spinal cord control and not enough brain control. Squeezing the hand will work the muscles to help reestablish brain control over those muscles. This will lead to less spasticity. If you choose this strategy also work on relaxing the hand. So you would first squeeze and then relax, squeeze, relax. To keep the fingernails from biting into the palm and also to practice this in different hand postures, squeeze an object. The classic example is a tennis ball. You can also use any number of squeeze toys or handgrip exercisers. Mix *repetitive practice into flexion* with a robust stretching program. The fingers should be stretched into the most possible non-painful extension of both the fingers and wrist at the same time ("prayer position").

Once repetitive practice provides enough movement, you can use constraint-induced therapy (see page 68) to take you the rest of the way.

WHAT PRECAUTIONS SHOULD BE TAKEN?

Any sort of repetitive practice takes a lot of effort. You are working your muscles and your brain in ways that are "new" (new since the stroke). Both your muscles and your brain are changing. This change requires a lot of energy. Fatigue can cause less focus on safety. Less focus on safety can lead to injury. And injury can stop recovery. Be sure you are well rested.

✳   ✳   ✳

IMAGINE IT!

Athletes do it. Musicians do it. Just about every motivational speaker recommends doing it. "It" is **mental practice** (MP)—also known as **imagery**. It has been used since the beginning of humankind to imagine an event before the event happens. This gives humans the unique ability to "practice" a task before it takes place. Although MP is done without actually moving, research has found that mental practice is *not* a passive process.

Mental practice, used alternately with actual practice, is an effective tool for recovery from stroke. It has the advantage of being easy, inexpensive, and safe, and it can be done almost anywhere.

Mental practice is actually an active process because:

- When you imagine moving your body, the muscles involved in those movements actually flex slightly, and they flex in the same pattern they do during the actual movement.
- When you move you use a particular portion of your brain to do those movements. When you do MP of those same movements, the same areas in the brain are used. Mental practice has been shown to rewire the brain after stroke. Studies have shown that mentally practicing something promotes as much neuroplastic change as actually practicing it!
- Mental practice is an active mental repetition of the task. Mental practice represents repeated attempts to imagine moving as one did prior to the stroke. Mental practice involves active, disciplined, and focused "mental attempts."

Immersive virtual reality (VR) has been shown to aid recovery after stroke (see You Are Game—Virtual Reality, page 87). Immersive VR involves a "wrap-around" experience; wherever you turn your head the virtual (artificial) environment is there. Mental practice resembles VR, but uses your mind instead of technology.

HOW IS IT DONE?

Mental practice has two elements to it:

- *Practicing the movement mentally.* The first thing to do is make an audio recording. The recording should first take you through a period of deep relaxation. The main idea during relaxation is to make yourself comfortable, empty the mind, and control breathing. The deep relaxation part of the tape should last 3 to 5 minutes.

Following deep relaxation is the actual MP portion of the recording. This portion will describe the task that will be mentally practiced. The recording should involve every aspect of the experience including the size of the room and full description of the movement, including the feel of the movement. It should sound something like, "Imagine you are sitting in your favorite chair. The room is quiet. There is a table in front of the chair...." Later, the details of the movement are filled in. "...imagine there is a cup on that table with fresh apple juice in it. Feel yourself reaching for the cup. Feel the weight of your arm as you reach out. Feel your elbow straightening and your wrist extending. Your hand opens, and your fingertips touch the cool china cup..." and so on.

It may be possible to do MP without the aid of an audio recording, but this has not been tested in research. Certainly athletes, musicians, and other performers use MP without audio recordings, so it may merit a try for stroke survivors as well. Just proceed through deep relaxation and then picture the movement. The more realistically you can imagine the task, the more effective the MP will be.

• *Practicing the movement in the real world.* Once the audio recording has been listened to a few times, practice the movement in reality. The ratio should be approximately three listening sessions to one actual practice session.

WHAT PRECAUTIONS SHOULD BE TAKEN?

Just because it is practiced "perfectly" does not mean it can actually be done perfectly. The reality is that the stroke survivor may or may not move better after mental practice. Therefore, if the stroke survivor is attempting to walk, it is necessary to understand the difference between the perfect movements imagined during mental practice sessions and the real-world realities of gravity, effort, and endurance.

✳   ✳   ✳

STIMULATE YOUR STRIDE

Stroke survivors often have difficulty lifting their foot at the ankle (**dor-siflexion**). This problem is called "drop foot" or "foot drop." Foot drop leads to what is essentially an ongoing series of trips unless a style of walking is used that raises the leg enough to have the foot safely clear the floor. There are four types of walking patterns stroke survivors typically use when they have foot drop:

- *Steppage gait* involves lifting the foot high off the ground by overly bending the knee in order to clear the floor.
- *Circumduction* involves sweeping the "bad" leg way out to the side so the foot can swing by.
- *Vaulting* involves raising the heel on the "good" leg in order to swing affected leg through.
- *Hip hiking* involves lifting the "bad" leg by using the muscles in the trunk to tilt the pelvis upward on the affected side, in order to let the "bad" leg swing through.

All of these styles of gait may bring a stroke survivor safely from point A to B. There is a downside to these sorts of unnatural walking patterns, however. Bone, cartilage, ligaments, and tendons work best during normal walking. The walking patterns often used after stroke cause stress on joints, the trunk, and back, which lead to arthritis and other disorders over time. More importantly, drop foot causes a gait that has the potential to lead to falls.

Doctors will prescribe an **ankle-foot orthosis** (**AFO**) for most stroke survivors who have drop foot. There are three good reasons to wear AFOs:

- They stabilize the ankle so it does not twist—a twisted ankle can lead to a fall.
- They allow walking to be safer.
- They make walking take less energy, so you can walk further.

But there is a downside to using AFOs. An AFO is used everyday and for the rest of your life. Because the AFO lifts the foot, you will never need to lift your foot again. Once the AFO is consistently used, several things can happen to the brain and muscles that can eliminate the chance of ever walking without an AFO again. Use of an AFO:

- Weakens the muscles that are normally used to lift the foot.

- Reduces the amount of brain dedicated to lifting the foot. A sort of reverse **neuroplasticity** occurs in the brain, so that the stroke survivor eventually loses any ability (or any future ability) to lift the foot on his or her own.
- Reduces **passive range of motion**. The ankle is rarely taken through its full natural range of motion because the AFO inhibits normal movement. The soft tissue surrounding the joints shortens, and passive range of motion is lost.

You can "jump start" the process of lifting your foot on your own again, however. There are special functional electrical stimulation (FES) systems that can reverse all the bad trends caused by AFOs. These FES systems increase quality of movement, range of motion, and strength, and make walking safe and effective. Research has shown that FES improves overall movement in the leg and improves walking ability.

HOW IS IT DONE?

There are muscles at the front of the lower leg, just to the outside of the shin bone, that lift the foot. These are the muscles that, when weakened by stroke, cause drop foot. Functional electrical stimulation systems provide low levels of electrical stimulation to the muscles that lift the foot while walking. Unlike an AFO, FES allows the stroke survivor's own muscles to actually do the work of lifting the foot. The stimulation is sent from a machine, either down a wire or through radio signals, into an electrode that lies against the skin just over the muscles and nerves that lift the foot. A doctor or therapist adjusts the system to obtain the best foot movement for the highest quality of walking.

Companies that make FES systems for walking include (in no particular order): NESS L300™, Odstock Dropped Foot Stimulator, and the WalkAide® System. Please note that all of these devices are outlined, with websites included, in the section entitled Recovery Machines (see page 169).

Functional electrical stimulation for walking may have more benefits than just helping you walk better. These systems may also:

- Strengthen muscles that are weak or paralyzed

- Stretch spastic muscles and other **soft tissue**
- Reduce spasticity
- Increase active range of motion
- Increase the amount of brainpower dedicated to lifting the foot

Some FES systems for drop foot cost about the same as a standard AFO. Some are much costlier. We can assume that the cost will steadily decrease because of competition and other market forces.

WHAT PRECAUTIONS SHOULD BE TAKEN?

This is not an off-the-shelf treatment. These systems require a prescription from a doctor and have to be fitted by a doctor or therapist. The stroke survivor needs specific training to start the therapy. The health-care workers involved in the process will detail all the necessary precautions.

❋   ❋   ❋

MIRROR THERAPY

During **mirror therapy** you use a mirror to reflect your "good" hand, while hiding your "bad" hand. The reflection of your unaffected hand makes it appear that both hands are moving normally. Researchers believe that seeing the reflection of the "good" hand tricks the brain into believing the affected hand is moving as well as the "good" hand. The mirror provides proper visual input so the brain can "remember" how the bad arm and hand *should* move. Mirror therapy provides the proper visual input because the reflection helps fool your brain into believing that your affected arm is moving correctly.

Most of the **neuroplastic** change outlined in this book involves reorganizing nerve cells in the area of the brain that controls movement. Mirror therapy may rewire cells in the sensory (feeling) part of the brain. Mirror therapy may restore the feeling of normal movement that has been missing since the stroke. This process may help improve limb movement. It is believed that the mirror creates positive reinforcement—because the affected

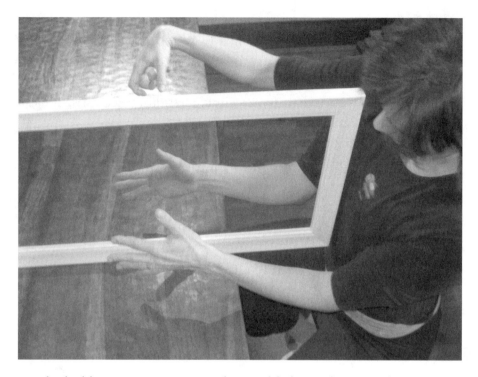

arm looks like it is moving correctly—and helps make a visual connection to muscle control, thereby strengthening the sensory-motor (feeling-moving) connection. This rewiring may help the affected limb move better.

HOW IS IT DONE?

Sit with the mirror facing the "good" side of your body. When you look in the mirror you will only see the "good" hand. You then practice moving both hands in the same way (symmetrically) at the same time, but only look at the unaffected hand.

Attempt to copy the movement of the "good" arm and hand with the "bad" arm and hand. The movements are done with both hands, at the same time. Here are examples of movements that can be tried:

- Opening and closing the hand
- Bending and straightening the wrist
- Touching the thumb to the fingertips

The affected hand attempts to make the same movement as the unaffected hand, like conducting an orchestra. Only look at the reflection of the good hand and make sure you cannot see the affected hand. Let the reflection of the "good" hand fool you into believing the affected hand is moving well. Typically this is done for 15-minute sessions, twice a day. You can use any freestanding mirror to do mirror therapy.

Reflex Pain Management Ltd. is a company that manufactures mirror boxes, which are perfect for mirror therapy. For further information contact:

- Reflex Pain Management Ltd
    Website: www.reflexpainmanagement.com.
    Email: mail@reflexpainmanagement.com

WHAT PRECAUTIONS SHOULD BE TAKEN?

Do not attempt this therapy with the lower extremity while standing. This lower-extremity therapy may be done with the legs and feet while lying down or seated.

✳   ✳   ✳

SPEAK MUSICALLY

The left side of the brain contains the language centers. Stroke on the left side of the brain may cause **aphasia** (trouble speaking or understanding what others are saying).

What if another area of the brain could take over for the damaged language portion of the brain? For instance, what if you could use a part of the *right* side of your brain for language? That is the aim of a therapy called **melodic intonation therapy** (MIT). This therapy uses a person's innate ability to process music in retraining the ability to speak after stroke. The right side of the brain is where music is perceived.

It is remarkable to hear someone who can barely talk, sing beautifully, with diction and word-finding in full bloom. This ability to use the intact "music portion" of the brain to communicate is one of the bright spots in emerging research on rehabilitation from aphasia. Melodic intonation therapy may be able to jump start the ability of the brain to rewire itself **neuroplastically**.

HOW IS IT DONE?

A speech therapist takes the stroke survivor through the process of retraining speech using MIT. This therapy may be effective in stroke survivors with certain deficits but who also have particular strengths. For instance, the best candidates for MIT are folks who:
- Can presently speak very little
- Can process sound correctly
- Understand when they make mistakes
- Are able to correct mistakes
- Are emotionally stable

Melodic intonation therapy involves exaggerating the sing-song aspect of speech. The stroke survivor is encouraged to express language as a series of tones, allowing words to form notes, and sentences to form melody. Imagine the song-like quality of children as they memorize a nursery rhyme, repeat their ABCs, or learn to count. This is much the same technique used to emphasize the pitch and rhythm of language. This may stimulate the right side of the brain to provide some of the power needed to speak.

WHAT PRECAUTIONS SHOULD BE TAKEN?

This therapy is done under the supervision of a speech therapist.

* * *

CONSTRAINT-INDUCED THERAPY FOR SPEECH

Constraint-induced therapy (CIT) in the arm and leg involves focusing the entire treatment on the "bad" side. In the upper extremity, the "good" arm and hand is constrained, usually with a sling or a mitt. This makes CIT in the arms relatively straightforward. In the leg, there is a problem because if you tie up the "good" leg, you're asking for trouble! Therapists handle the challenge of using CIT in the leg by overloading the leg with large amounts of safe exercises. Constraint-induced therapy for **expressive aphasia**, called constraint-induced aphasia therapy (CIAT) shares many of the same techniques used in arms and legs.

HOW IS IT DONE?

All of the constraint therapies require :

- *Hours per day of focused and dedicated practice* for between 2-3 weeks
  — CIT: Between 5-7 hours a day of movement practice.
  — CIAT: Delivered with schedules of 2-3 hours a day. Research indicates that this level of intensity is necessary to rewire the language areas of the brain.
- *Forcing the stroke survivors to work on their weakness*
  — CIT: Uses a sling or mitt to constrain the "good" hand
  — CIAT: Prevents non-verbal communication including hand gestures, writing, and drawing
- *Repetition of desired behavior*
  — CIT: Movements are practiced over and over
  — CIAT: Sounds, words, and sentences are repeated.
- *Constant challenge*
  — CIT: Movements attempted are made difficult over time
  — CIAT: More difficult sounds, words, and sentence structures are attempted over time

For better speech to occur, intense, focused, and repeated attempts have to be made. This will provide new pathways for neurons (nerve cells) in the brain to navigate around the area in the brain that died during the stroke. These pathways become stronger with each repetition and end up "hard wiring" to each other, allowing the stroke survivor to speak better.

In some ways CIAT is designed to do exactly the opposite of what stroke survivors with aphasia tend to do naturally. Here are some examples:

- Folks who are aphasic tend to not speak much because they feel that communicating may not be worth the effort. They often simply stop trying to talk at all or give up in the middle of sentences. Constraint-induced aphasia therapy does not allow *not* talking, or abandoning what you want to say. In fact, it forces hours of speaking a day.

- Folks who are aphasic tend to use other forms of communication, things like gesturing, tone of voice on a single repeated word, or writing. This is where the constraint part of constraint-induced aphasia therapy comes in. During CIAT you are not allowed to communicate in any way that does not involve talking.

Constraint-induced aphasia therapy is done under the supervision of a speech therapist. Constraint therapies tend to be expensive because of the large amount of clinical hours involved. Insurance does not typically pay for CIT and CIAT. Of course, just like many of the ideas in this book, certain elements of CIAT can be done on your own. There are elements of all the constraint therapies, including CIAT that you can adopt and make part of your recovery effort. Repetition of sounds, words, and sentences and focused, dedicated practice can be done at home to augment what you learn with your speech therapist.

WHAT PRECAUTIONS SHOULD BE TAKEN?

Consult you doctor prior to starting this therapy. Constraint-induced aphasia therapy is nothing if not vigorous, and the health implications of the effort and frustrations inherent in relearning to talk may have global health implications.

✳　　✳　　✳

YOU ARE GAME—VIRTUAL REALITY

Virtual reality (VR) has the potential to make recovery fun while being safe and challenging. You can become involved in the game either by wearing a VR mask or goggles, or by looking at a TV or computer screen. While playing, you are physically challenged. For instance, a game may ask the player to "catch" a virtual ball or use a plastic saber to slay characters on the screen. The great thing about VR is that you can challenge yourself in new and imaginative ways, safely seated in the most comfortable chair in your home.

People love video games because they are designed to have an interesting and realistic look. They are fun, competitive, and challenging. Many people look at video games as passive entertainment. But for the stroke survivor, virtual-reality technologies provide a physical challenge that has one strong advantage over real-world rehabilitation: safety. With video games, you can walk, run, and ski... perform almost any activity within the safety of an armchair. Stroke survivors can use VR to help develop better balance, better arm and hand movement, and increased strength. Unfortunately, much of stroke recovery can be boring. Many repetitions of a movement are needed to rewire the brain so that movement is improved. But repetitive movement, done thousands of times, is not the most interesting way to spend your time. This is especially true because, during recovery from stroke, you are not learning new and exciting skills. You are simply relearning skills that you did perfectly prior to your stroke. Virtual reality allows repetitive practice to occur while using your own natural sense of competition and creativity in an engaging 3-D environment. In short, VR makes repetitive practice fun.

HOW IS IT DONE?

These gaming systems are available in toy stores for under $50. The fact that many of the games are inexpensive allows you to be creative while managing your own recovery. Use games that are challenging, fun, and maintain safety.

Virtual-reality technology can be an effective way of increasing **active movement** in the hands and arms after stroke. The trick is finding a game that will challenge the hand and arm in a way that is interesting and fun. Therapies that engage you tend to be more productive so make sure the game is interesting to you. Make sure the game challenges you in a way that promotes recovery. Using virtual reality as a recovery tool can be as simple as a joystick. For instance, if you decide that you need help with small amounts of elbow flexion, extension, pronation, and supination (turning the hand palm up and down), then a joystick might be the perfect recovery tool. Many of these games are "plug and play" so that they plug right into your TV. However, VR that is immersive is more effective than games played on flat screens. Immersive means that you are wearing a head-mounted display or 3-D glasses. As you turn your head, you are completely sur-rounded by the visual experience.

WHAT PRECAUTIONS SHOULD BE TAKEN?

Virtual reality may not be a safe option for balance exercises in some stroke survivors. However, leg exercises can be made safe by using your legs to play the game while you are sitting. For instance if the game asks you to kick a ball, make sure you can accomplish this while sitting in a chair.

Just like any exercise, virtual reality should be done within the recom-mendations of your doctor. Discontinue any exercise if it causes pain. Be-cause VR is engaging, you might be less aware of discomfort or safety issues. It is prudent to consult with a therapist prior to using rehabilitation gaming so that the training is effective and safe.

✳   ✳   ✳

RHYTHM REHAB FOR THE ARMS AND HANDS

It's a cliché that many people have heard: "Rhythm is essential to life." Everything you do, from the grand cycles of life and death, to the pulse of heartbeat and the pattern of breathing, is rhythmic. There is power in rhythm that can be used to recover from stroke. Some aspects of recovery are natu-rally rhythmic. Walking and stationary cycling movements are rhythmic, but both are lower-extremity exercises. Setting up challenges that involve rhythm for the upper extremity requires a little creativity and ingenuity.

You need some sort of machine to provide a beat. This can be a metronome, which is a machine that musicians use to keep a constant rhythm. Inexpensive metronomes cost about $10. Most electronic keyboards, which usually have some sort of beat-keeping mechanism built in, can be used. Of course, the easiest way to involve a beat in recovery is listening to music. As long as the music has a constant beat, music will work. Music has an added advantage: it takes your mind off the fatigue factor. There is a rea-son that most exercise videos involve music; listening to music provides a distraction from the difficulty of the exercise. This is the same reason that so many runners listen to music and the reason music headsets are banned from many running races. It is believed that the music actually provides an unfair benefit to people listening to music during strenuous athletic events.

Music may have the added benefit of providing motivation. Nothing motivates people like their favorite music. Music can become the soundtrack of your life that, just like in movies, adds color to recovery efforts.

HOW IS IT DONE?

Here is a simple way a beat can be used to help the "good" arm/hand to train the "bad" arm/hand:

- Place two towels on a table.
- Measure how far the "bad" hand can reach while sliding on the towel across the table. Make sure the affected elbow is at its fullest extension (most straight) and your back is against the seat back. Place a piece of tape at the furthest point you can reach, directly in front of the hand. Repeat the process for the "good" hand.

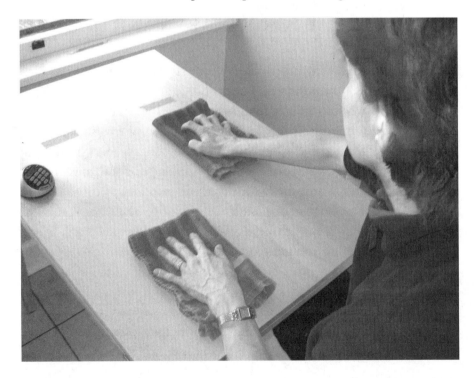

- Sit at the table so that one hand and wrist is on each towel. Keep your back against the seat back.
- Set the metronome so you can hit the targets on clicks. With each successive click, have first your unaffected hand and then your affected hand push the towel forward until the tape target is met.
- As one hand is going forward, the other goes back, in alternating motion.
- Increase the speed of the beat or the distance reached to increase challenge.

The same basic rules would apply to any exercise you devise. Simply follow these guidelines:

- Make targets equal for both hands and arms. The targets don't have to be on a table. For instance, you could have each hand reaching as high a point as the "bad" arm can reach.
- Set a challenging rhythmic rate.
- Set a timer so you know when to start and when to stop. If you use music, use the length of the song or piece as the start and stop points.
- Keep the rhythm!

WHAT PRECAUTIONS SHOULD BE TAKEN?

Special emphasis should be placed on the possibility of spikes in blood pressure and pulse rate because this type of therapy can increase both.

For the upper extremities, this is a relatively safe technique, but again, if used for walking, marching, or anything that involves balance, be extra cautious, and consult your physician and physical therapist.

✳   ✳   ✳

RHYTHM REHAB FOR THE LEG

Physical therapists focus on the mechanics of gait (how the legs and feet are used during walking). There is another important aspect to walking that gets less attention: rhythm. Walking after a stroke is often like bicycling on two square tires; there is a lack of a predictable rhythm. Researchers have successfully used what is called **rhythmic auditory cuing** to revive proper rhythm during walking. Any sort of rhythmic movement in the legs, arms, or a combination of all four limbs can benefit from this technique. This may even be worth a try with expressive aphasia. If words come out slowly, matching words to an increasing rhythm may accelerate the rate at which words can be formed. Using rhythm for recovery in the legs involves listening to and matching a beat while you walk. This can help reestablish the natural rhythm of gait. Since the main function of the legs is to walk, developing a good and natural rhythm will help gait look and feel smoother and more symmetrical.

HOW IS IT DONE?

This sort of auditory cuing is simply a constant "click," like the ticking of a clock. In research experiments, a metronome (a device that musicians use to keep time while practicing their instruments) is used. Metronomes can be purchased for less than $10. Any device that produces a constant and predictable beat can be used. As long as the speed of the beat can be altered, a drum machine, a keyboard with programmable beats, or a metronome can be used. Music can be used as well. The company Biodex has a treadmill specifically designed to provide audio feedback to encourage symmetry in walking (see Recovery Machines, page 169).

The trick is finding a constant rhythm that is close to the rhythm of the movement being done. Researchers have often found it difficult to have patients match the beat of music precisely during walking. This therapy can be done while marching in place and while holding on to something strong, solid, and immobile. A wall-mounted bar or a sturdy chair may provide the necessary element of safety while marching in place. During treadmill walking, rhythm can be used to establish the rhythm of footfalls.

When the foot hits the ground (cadence) can be sped up or slowed down by changing the length of your steps. Shortening steps will speed up cadence, and lengthening steps will slow down cadence.

This concept of using rhythm to help the timing of movement may also help in other ways. Experiments have shown that people who run while listening to music feel less fatigue than those who don't listen to music. The same may be true with stroke survivors. Music can provide a hypnotic escape from an otherwise boring exercise routine.

WHAT PRECAUTIONS SHOULD BE TAKEN?

The lower extremities of stroke survivors are notoriously hard to lock into a beat. The differences in strength and coordination between the "good" and "bad" sides make keeping a constant and steady beat while walking near impossible. Even for folks who have not had a stroke, walking in perfect rhythm is difficult. There is a reason that the military spends so much time having soldiers walk in rhythm; it's hard to do. For this reason the following recommendation exists:

Do not do this sort of rhythmic training while standing or walking without the recommendation of your doctor and the guidance of physical and/or occupational therapy staff.

*   *   *

THE GOOD TRAINS THE BAD— BILATERAL TRAINING

Most of the movements people do are **bilateral** (using either the two upper or the two lower limbs working together). Even the movements that you think are done with just one limb involve the other limb without you even thinking about it. Consider handwriting with a pencil (or pen) and paper. It turns out that the nonwriting hand has an important role in shifting the paper. Handwriting will get much slower and sloppier if the nonwriting hand is not involved. Another example is threading a needle. It would be easy to believe that if the needle was held steady in a vise that it would be easier to thread because the needle would be held perfectly stationary. Yet when someone encounters this situation, the first instinct is to hold the needle. It turns out that when a person threads a needle, both hands are involved in an intricate and effective dance to get the needle threaded as efficiently as possible.

For folks who have *not* had a stroke, research has shown something remarkable: when both hands are used together in tasks, the movement of the non-dominant hand (in most of us the left hand) improves movement quality, accuracy, and speed. Researchers have found a similar dynamic in stroke survivors. When the "good" arm and "bad" arm are doing the same movements at the same time, the "bad" arm moves better. This is also true when the two arms do equal and opposite movements. When the two limbs are moved together, the movement in the affected limb improves its movement quality and movement accuracy. Using **bilateral training** helps the unaffected side train the affected side. In the leg, walking provides automatic bilateral training. Since you can't walk with one leg, the "bad" leg is forced to work, bilaterally, with the "good" leg. This may be one reason that the leg tends to recover faster than the arm. The arm and hand also benefit from this sort of training, but recovery efforts have to be specifically set up to allow for this type of training in the arm and hand.

HOW IS IT DONE?

The best way to allow for bilateral training of the arm and hands is to promote movement where the two extremities do the same (or equal) but opposite movements. The arm will follow what the hand attempts, so the hand will be the primary focus in the following exercises.

Bilateral training can take two forms:

- Equal and at the same time: the two hands can work in unison (the same movement at the same time, as in a mirror image):
  — Throwing a two-handed basketball pass
  — Folding clothes symmetrically
  — Pretending to conduct an orchestra to classical music
  — Drumming both hands at the same time (add challenge by playing to music)
  — Placing objects (blocks, cups, cones) close to you and then away from you at the same time
  — Spooning out dry ingredients with both hands at the same time

- Equal and alternating (reciprocal): The two hands can work in equal opposition (each arm and hand does equal but opposite movements):
  — Alternate punching
  — Drumming
  — Asymmetrical cloth folding
  — Hand-over-hand rope pulling
  — Alternating wiping of a table with a towel
  — Tapping a target while alternating hands
  — Tapping a balloon from one hand to the other (add difficulty by tossing a ball from one hand to the other)

The possibilities are endless. All of these can be done to a rhythm (see Rhythm Rehab for the Arms and Hands, page 89), which will make you focus on equal movement done during equal amounts of time. The rhythm in music or the constant click of a metronome can be used to make the two limbs do the task within the same time limits.

All of the previously listed suggestions involve the arms and hands, but similar exercises can be performed with the legs and feet. With the leg and foot, the rules are the same as the arm and hand: whatever movement one leg does, the other matches (equal and at the same time, and equal and alternating).

The more you match the movements of the "good" limb, the better. If you find matching the two limbs is too easy, add difficulty by adding speed. That is, accelerate the movement of the "good" limb, and try to continue to match the movement with the "bad" limb. Rhythmic movements with the legs and feet can be done while lying on the back, sitting, or in a recumbent position.

WHAT PRECAUTIONS SHOULD BE TAKEN?

Most of these exercises can be done in a seated position with little or no significant risk. If any of these exercises are done in a standing position, added stress is put on balance, leg strength, and stamina. For this reason, do not perform this sort of bilateral training while standing without the recommendation of your doctor and the guidance of a physical and/or occupational therapy staff.

✳   ✳   ✳

SHOCKING SUBLUXATION

When someone has a stroke, there is often a period of time when the muscles on the affected side are completely limp (flaccid). During this stage of recovery, there is no muscle activity. Even basic reflexes that keep muscles tight (spastic) in later **stages of recovery** are not present. Muscles are usually flaccid right after the stroke, but flaccid muscles can continue for years. When the muscles that hold the shoulder joint in place are flaccid, the shoulder will dislocate. In stroke survivors, shoulder dislocation is called **subluxation of the shoulder**.

The shoulder is an unusual joint. It is called a ball-in-socket joint, but should be called a "ball-on-a-flat-surface joint." Unlike other four-limbed animals, humans have developed arms (called forelimbs in animals) that have a huge **range of motion** at the shoulder. This has given humans the ability to move their hands around in a wide area, which gives them the ability to do everything from throwing to climbing.

But humans pay a price for this great movement: the shoulder joint is relatively weak. The joint is formed by one round surface (the round top or "head" of the bone that makes up the upper arm) and a flat area, which is part of the shoulder blade. The shoulder joint is held together rather weakly by muscles that surround the joint. If these shoulder muscles become either weak or paralyzed, the weight of the arm pulls the joint apart. In some stroke survivors, the shoulder muscles reawaken as recovery continues, and the shoulder joint is pulled back into proper alignment. In other stroke survivors shoulder subluxation can continue for years.

Along with the naturally weak human shoulder joint and the increased weakness of the joint after stroke, stroke survivors have an added risk: well-meaning people pulling on their affected arm. During transfers (i.e., sitting to standing, lying down to sitting, etc.) it is common for health-care workers or caregivers to use the affected side arm to pull the stroke survivor into position. Ouch!

When a muscle is completely flaccid after stroke, only one thing can make it contract: electrical stimulation (**e-stim**). This treatment is called **neuromuscular electrical stimulation** (**NMES**). NMES machines can provide e-stim into the muscles that surround the shoulder joint. When the stimulation enters the muscle, the muscle contracts and pulls the top arm bone (humerus) into position. The e-stim actually contracts (tightens) the muscles, in much the same way the stroke survivor would, if they could. In this way, the electrical stimulation, over time, can strengthen the muscles surrounding the shoulder joint. For some stroke survivors, this helps normal muscle activity hold the joint together permanently.

HOW IS IT DONE?

The electrodes are placed on the deltoid and supraspinatus muscles. These muscles are located on the side and the top of the shoulder. Many machines on the market can provide electrical stimulation, in the proper dose, to resolve subluxation. A doctor's order and a therapist's guidance will establish the best electrode placement and type of stimulation parameters.

Percutaneous (performed through the skin) **intramuscular stimulation** (perc-NMES) is another option. This form of stimulation is much like NMES, but the electrodes are placed directly into the weakened muscles. This allows for less e-stim needed because there is less tissue between the stimulation source (the machine) and the stimulation target (the muscles). Perc-NMES also has the advantage of being able to more accurately target the specific muscles that can help reduce subluxation. This treatment involves minor surgery.

Note that NMES is different from the form of e-stim that is often used clinically, called transcutaneous electrical nerve stimulation (TENS) often used to reduce pain, even the pain of subluxation. The TENS sort of e-stim does not make the muscle contract, and so would be ineffective in reducing subluxation.

WHAT PRECAUTIONS SHOULD BE TAKEN?

Your doctor will let you know if this therapy will be effective and safe for you. There are some contraindications for e-stim because the electrical output can interfere with other electrical devices (i.e., pacemakers). Always consult your doctor before attempting this therapy. Have your occupational or physical therapist help you decide how and where the stimulation should be used. Once your doctor and therapist are consulted, e-stim may be able to be administered with an inexpensive machine, at home.

Elements of Exercise Essential to Recovery

GET A HOME EXERCISE PROGRAM

Being able to depend on physical, occupational, and speech therapists for ongoing therapy is an ideal situation. Therapists provide knowledge, guidance, and encouragement. Unfortunately therapists, and the facilities where therapists work, are expensive. Insurance will only pay for a certain amount of therapy. So what's a stroke survivor to do?

A home exercise program (HEP) is the group of exercises that the therapist gives you to do at home after all the therapy sessions are over. These exercises are usually given right before being discharged from therapy. The HEP may be provided before **discharge** from the hospital, again just before discharge from any skilled nursing facility, again during outpatient therapy, and then again at the end of any home therapy.

Therapists tend to leave the review of HEP until the final few visits, and the HEP usually is simply a rehash of the exercises done with the therapist during the course of therapy. Stroke survivors are handed a few photocopies of pictures or descriptions of exercises, and a review of those exercises is done. Here's a little a joke for this process:

"What does HEP stand for?"

"Hand 'Em Photocopies."

But there is a problem with this traditional view of the HEP. Making a lifelong plan toward recovery is essential to maximizing potential. Unfortunately, therapists, who are in the best position to develop a long-term recovery plan, often take a short-sighted view of the HEP and generally treat it as an afterthought, discussed right before the end of therapy. Home exercise programs developed by therapists tend to be rigid, reflecting only what is on the photocopied pages. This casual view is not only short sighted, it is actually detrimental to any further recovery. The traditional view of a HEP promotes the assumption that the stroke survivor won't get any better. This is a built-in self-fulfilling prophecy: the same exercises that were used in therapy, the same exercises that did not promote progress (but did achieve **plateau**) and triggered the end of therapies will, at best, retain the present level of strength, coordination, and ability. The thinking is, "Since the system has determined that the stroke survivor won't improve, she should keep doing the same thing." The typical HEP has no built-in points at which it should be updated and no flexibility to help promote progress toward recovery.

The problem with the perspective of some therapists is that their experience has told them that any given stroke survivor will make nominal progress after he ends treatment, and this is evident from a purely statistical standpoint; most patients either do not progress or actually get worse after discharge from therapy. But if you take the advice in this book, recovery should continue until you have reached your maximum potential. This willingness to go beyond what traditional stroke rehabilitation has to offer will be an unusual view to most therapists, so you may have to coach them through the process. For instance, perhaps you are not walking upon discharge from all therapies. But after you are discharged, you start a new leg-strengthening program that allows you to take a few steps. What do you do now? How do you build on this progress? How do you develop the cardiovascular stamina to walk farther? Which muscles should you stretch, and which should you strengthen to facilitate more walking?

Let therapists know that what is required is a strategy that will help you to continue to make *gains*. Ask them to build into a HEP the flexibility that will constantly provide higher goals, and ask therapists to provide the tools and strategies to achieve those goals. These requests are going to challenge therapists in ways that they are not usually challenged, and you may get some strange looks. But remember, you are paying (and paying well) for therapy, and having them provide an adequate and challenging home exercise program is well within their job description.

Also, challenge your physiatrist and therapists with suggestions of techniques and technologies that you find during your research. If you see something that you think would work, ask them to follow through by explaining and implementing that therapy. Remember: You were most likely discharged because these health professionals believed that you have **plateaued** (not going to get any better). If therapists just continue to use the same techniques then, indeed, you will not get any better. Why? Because the same techniques will probably continue to get the same results. In your own attempts toward recovery, look for new therapies that might work, and have doctors and therapists implement the therapies. Stroke survivors and friends and families are the best advocates!

HOW IS IT DONE?

A HEP that includes effective therapeutic interventions and exercises is essential to ongoing recovery from stroke. Here are some suggestions when consulting with a therapist about the HEP:

- Start planning your HEP with your therapists as early as possible. Tell therapists you work with, from the hospital to home therapy, to provide the information and tools needed to continue progress at home.
- Let therapists know that you want a strategy that will help you continue to make significant gains, not retain existing levels of performance.
- Ask therapists to build flexibility into the HEP, so that it will constantly provide higher goals, and ask therapists to give you tools and strategies to achieve those goals.
- Repeat these steps as time goes on. Every year or so (more if it's needed, less if you continue to make great gains on your own) go back through the cycle of seeing the **physiatrist** and any appropriate therapists so that they can help you tweak your HEP. This will ensure that your at-home work continues to be challenging and fruitful.

The last week or so before ending therapies is way too late to work with therapists to develop a HEP. The HEP should be developed, in a rolling manner, from the beginning of your relationship with therapists. These professionals are trained to develop plans toward recovery. Much of their education is dedicated to the development of these sorts of plans. Many therapists end sessions because they are forced to by pressure from managed care (insurance companies). Most will be happy that you want to continue to make progress once your relationship with them ends. But unless you prod and prompt therapists, and provide adequate time toward this goal, they will take the traditional perspective and wait until the last few days to "Hand 'Em Photocopies."

The best way to plan for a fruitful "rest of your life" after discharge is to make it clear to the occupational, physical, and speech therapists that you take your recovery very seriously, and you know that recovery will continue long after you've forgotten their names.

WHAT PRECAUTIONS SHOULD BE TAKEN?

The HEP will be implemented when the therapist is no longer around. This may add to the therapist's reluctance to develop a HEP beyond what you've done in his or her care; they don't want to plan anything new that may put you into danger. Agree with him or her prior to the development of the HEP that you will take any safety precautions seriously, and you will inform your doctor as you progress. Anytime you significantly alter your exercise or therapy routine, inform your doctor. The doctor will agree and encourage your ongoing efforts 99% of the time. But let the doctor make the final decision about the safety of the program.

As elements are added to the HEP, be sensitive to changes inherent in your body and mind. If you feel that something is hurting you or is too strenuous, stop. Generally, pain can be trusted as a warning of something significantly harmful.

✳ ✳ ✳

SPACE TO RECOVER—THE HOME GYM

Clearly, it's easier to study at the library, do paperwork at your desk, and cook in the kitchen. Every stroke survivor also needs a space within his or her home dedicated to recovery. It should be a space where you can focus on recovering from your stroke. Like a library, it should only have the distractions you want; like a desk, it should be organized; like a kitchen, it should have all the recovery tools you need. It can be a basement, an extra bedroom, or a corner of a room.

Some stroke survivors prefer to peruse at least some of their recovery effort in a community gym. Even if one joins a community gym (see Space To Focus—The Community Gym, page 104), there are great reasons for having a home gym as well.

HOW IS IT DONE?

Your home gym does not have to be big and does not have to have any more equipment than you need. Your home gym should have what is necessary to facilitate recovery. This may include exercise equipment, a TV, VCR, DVD player, a stereo, and inspirational art. Build your gym as a place of sanctuary and a place of work. Ideas for equipment include:

- A treadmill
- A recumbent cycle
- An upper body ergometer (handcycle)
- An exercise mat
- Parallel bars or other equipment used to maintain balance
- Weights
- Resistance bands
- Electrical stimulation devices
- Balls, decks of cards, or other "toys"

This list can be as long or as short as it needs to be. A small amount of simple equipment that is well thought out and well used is better than a lot of expensive equipment left in a corner. The list of needed equipment can be added to with the help of doctors and therapists.

WHAT PRECAUTIONS SHOULD BE TAKEN?

Be prudent when assembling the gym and think safety first. Any exercise or therapy equipment has inherent dangers. For instance, a treadmill provides a moving surface that may be inappropriate for some stroke survivors. Even something as simple as a ball can facilitate a loss of balance that can cause a fall. Consider installing grab-bars for any balance exercises you do. Make sure the floor is non-slip given the footwear you expect to use. Doctors will tell you if an exercise or therapy is safe, and therapists will explain how to do the exercise or therapy in the most effective way possible.

*   *   *

SPACE TO FOCUS—THE COMMUNITY GYM

A community gym is a great place to focus on recovery. A well-equipped gym, with a supportive staff, provides the environment needed to build muscle, stamina, and flexibility. Gyms often have a pool. Pools provide the buoyancy and resistance of water to aid in recovery. Treadmills, weights, exercise balls, saunas, even giant mirrors, which provide valuable visual feedback, are usually available at the local gym. Gyms are motivating because motivated people go to them. Just being around other folks trying to reach their goals can be motivating.

Gyms in your community are not equipped the same as a home gym. Your home gym will have equipment that is specific to your recovery. For instance, your home gym might have an **e-stim** machine, a pegboard, or a deck of cards; all essential to your recovery but not available at any gym. The role that the community gym plays in your recovery is different from the role of your home gym. The community gym will be a place of "the big three" of exercise: cardiovascular training, weight training, and stretching, even though you might also do any or all of these at home. These types of exercises are essential aspects of recovery in order to "bank" the energy needed for every other part of the recovery effort.

Some stroke survivors actually get in better shape *after* their stroke than they were before their stroke. This may happen for several reasons, including:

- A new emphasis on staying in shape
- A new emphasis on diet
- More exercise
- More time available to exercise

The gym experience is a central part of life after stroke for some stroke survivors. Gyms can be centers of social contact and relaxation. Gyms can be exciting places if you are motivated. Gyms can also help you focus if you are less than motivated. Gyms provide a great combination of assets to help on the road to recovery.

HOW IS IT DONE?

A gym that is appropriate for recovery from stroke will have:

- Appropriate gear
- Surroundings in which the stroke survivor feels comfortable and relaxed
- A knowledgeable and supportive staff

Personnel at gyms do not often have expertise about, or experience with, folks with disabilities. Differences in credentialling add to the confusion. You should know that:

- Athletic trainers have a bachelor's degree in athletic training and are certified by the State in which they practice.
- Personal trainers need no education and no certification.

There are many stories of stroke survivors receiving the wrong advice from well-meaning gym employees. Have a physical and/or occupational therapist direct the rehab program. They don't have to go to the gym with you. The PT and/or OT simply needs to know what equipment is available so they can set up a safe and effective program. Of course, it would be highly beneficial if the therapist could go to the gym to direct the first session!

Try to find a gym that is close to where you live, and try to incorporate as much of the trip to the gym as possible into your lifestyle. That is, if you can find a gym that you can walk to, use the walking as part of your recovery. If you don't have a gym that close, at least make it convenient to your home or place of work.

Finding a gym whose members reflect your age group and gender will help you feel comfortable. Before joining a gym, tour the facility during the time that you would usually go. This will help determine the makeup of the membership and will help determine how crowded it might be during the time that you would typically go. Try to find a gym that offers classes that may facilitate stroke recovery. While spinning or rock climbing may not be within your interest and capacity, yoga, Tai Chi, or water aerobics may fit your ability and goals. Accessibility may be an issue as well. It is the law (within the Americans with Disabilities Act or ADA) that businesses must provide wheelchair accessible entrances, exits, and bathrooms. This may not be the case, however. Most gyms make the effort to comply. But some of the equipment may not be accessible for folks with an inability to walk or transfer (i.e., get on/off equipment). For instance, a hydraulic lift chair is available in many pools to safely transfer folks with mobility problems in and out of a pool. But many pools do not have one, so consider this when choosing a gym.

Your insurance may be willing to pay for some or all of your gym membership.

WHAT PRECAUTIONS SHOULD BE TAKEN?

Inform your doctor before starting or changing any exercise program.

✻   ✻   ✻

WEIGHT UP!

Resistance training is the general term for any exercise in which muscles work against resistance. The most common type of resistance training is weight training (sometimes called weight lifting). Resistance training provides many important benefits to a post-stroke therapy routine. Taken in total, these benefits make resistance training essential in any serious efforts toward recovery from stroke.

Resistance training and weight training are sometimes used interchangeably. For clarification, here are the distinctions:

- *Resistance training*: Resistance training is pushing (or pulling) against an opposing force. This includes your own resistance (e.g., pushing one hand against the other), someone else's resistance, gravity, resistance bands (made from sheets of rubber or rubber tubing), etc.
- *Weight training*: Weight training is resistance training where the force against which you are pushing (or pulling) is weights, which include barbells, dumbbells, and weight machines (like those found in a gym).

This chapter uses the more catch-all term *resistance training*. Here is a list of reasons to add this sort of training to your daily routine:

Resistance training:
- Increases strength on the "good" and "bad" side
- Improves mobility (walking, wheelchair movement, etc.)
- Reverses muscle atrophy (muscles getting smaller and weaker). Atrophy affects both the affected and unaffected side after stroke.
- Increases functional ability. ("Functional" is a buzz word used by health-care workers that describes the ability to do normal, everyday activities. Also known as ADLs or activities of daily living).

• Increases strength, which helps all other efforts toward recovery

Bone density is an important benefit of weight training because the denser a bone is, the stronger it is. There is a process that happens in bones called **Wolf's law**. Wolf's law says that a bone will get thicker and stronger because of the stresses that are put on it. As muscle pulls on bone, the bone responds by getting thicker. Over time, the more stress on the bone by the muscles, the greater the bone growth. Resistance training increases bone density.

Wolf's law works in the opposite way as well. The less stress that is put on bones the thinner bones get. After stroke, the muscles on the weak side contract (tighten) less. Thus, the affected side muscles put less stress on the affected side bones so there is less bone growth. Because you tend to fall toward the weak side (the side which has thinner bones) you are at a much greater risk of fracture. Increasing bone thickness on the "bad" side with resistance training reduces the chance of fracture.

There are other benefits to weight training that are not specific to stroke survivors but are important to everyone's health. (Keep in mind that diabetes, obesity, and high blood pressure are risk factors for stroke.) Resistance training:

• Helps to balance blood sugar, which is important for diabetics and pre-diabetics
• Increases resting metabolism, which reduces weight or reduces the speed at which weight is gained
• Reduces blood pressure

HOW IS IT DONE?

Resistance training helps with so many of the body's systems that it is good for everyone. But for folks who have had a stroke, resistance training is doubly important. Incorporate resistance training into a stroke-recovery strategy and be prepared for increases in energy, muscle strength, and endurance.

When deciding where resistance training fits into your recovery plan, carefully consider what area of the body to focus on. The recovery plan should include resistance training for all four limbs as well as your trunk (the area from mid-chest to hips, including the back). But some muscle groups will receive more focus than others. For instance, if it has been determined that walking will benefit from resistance training of the quadriceps (the large front thigh muscles that extend the knee and help flex the hip) then that's where more time and resistance training should be put. Accurately evaluating which muscles need work is the first step in developing your resistance training program. Therapists can help you determine which muscles need the most work. You can also help determine what muscles to work on using common sense and intuition. Generally speaking, stroke survivors have much less weakness in the flexor muscles than the extensor muscles. Flexor muscles are muscles that decrease joint angles. For instance, in the elbow, the flexor muscles bend the elbow. The extensor muscles straighten the elbow. The elbow well exemplifies the problem that stroke survivors typically have: They can bend the elbow pretty well, but cannot straighten the elbow. This is a case where resistance training would be better directed toward the extensor muscles than the flexors muscles. Focus on muscle groups (groups of muscles that work together) that are weakest. There will be a tendency to work muscle groups that are easily moved and somewhat less affected by the stroke. See Challenge Equals Recovery, page 22, for strategies to focus on what is hardest. This is not to say that the stronger of the two muscle groups, the flexors, should not be worked as well. Despite the fact that the flexor muscles tend to overpower, both sets of muscles are weak after stroke. But most of resistance training should be directed toward the extensor muscles muscle group, which tends to be the weakest after stroke.

It is not necessary to buy expensive equipment to add resistance training to your recovery effort. The following work just as well as expensive weights or weight machines:

- Elastic bands or cords
- The force of your own body against itself (isometric exercise, e.g., grasping the fingers of one hand with the other hand and pulling both hands away from each other)
- The force of gravity (e.g., squats, heel-ups, press-ups)

When deciding how to incorporate resistance training into a recovery plan keep in mind the following:

- Consult your doctor and therapist. They will help you determine the exercises that should be done, the progression of those exercises, and the equipment needed.

- Proper progression of exercises, to keep muscles challenged while maintaining safety, is an essential part of resistance training. Progression of resistance training should involve, over an arc of time, an increase in the number of repetitions, an increase of resistance (weight), or both.

WHAT PRECAUTIONS SHOULD BE TAKEN?

Start resistance training slowly and allow for a gradual progression. There is a phenomenon called "delayed-onset muscle soreness," commonly known as "DOMS." When DOMS does occur, this muscular soreness is felt from a day to a few days after the resistance training. This is a good reason to start slowly and evaluate how your muscles feel often. Building muscle involves developing small tears in muscle fibers, so a small amount of muscular pain is to be expected. The muscle is "repaired" by coming back thicker and stronger.

Consult you doctor regarding any health risks that may occur because of resistance training. Your doctor will tell you how the medications you are taking may affect your body's response to exercise. Have your occupational or physical therapist help you design a resistance training program that is safe, has built-in increases of challenges over time, and is appropriate to your particular deficits and personal goals. Take blood pressure and pulse rate before, during, and after resistance training (see Five Tests You Should Do, page 62). Some doctors may not want resistance training incorporated if the stroke survivor has had a hemorrhagic stroke (bleeding stroke) because of the risk of another stroke due to possible spikes in blood pressure during resistance training.

$$*\quad*\quad*$$

BANK ENERGY AND WATCH YOUR INVESTMENT GROW

Cardiovascular, also known as cardiorespiratory, fitness refers to the ability of the heart, blood vessels, and lungs to supply oxygen to muscles during exercise. Stroke survivors face unique challenges when it comes to their cardiovascular strength.

- Stroke survivors have *half* the amount of stamina as age-matched, out-of-shape "couch potatoes."
- It takes stroke survivors *twice* the amount of energy to do many daily activities like walking.

So, there is less energy available and more energy needed. This is why stamina exercise and weight training (muscle building, see Weight Up!, page 107) are so important. There is a reason athletes start their season with physically demanding workouts. They are banking energy for the game itself. You should do the same. Basic forms of exercise provide the stamina that's needed to pursue the other challenges of recovery. You can bank energy by following a challenging and safe cardiovascular exercise program. *Cardiovascular stamina (along with muscular strength) is the foundation on which every other effort toward recovery is built.* It's that simple. Strength of conviction and inner strength can be sky high, but if you don't have the other kinds of strength you are stopped before you begin. On the other hand, if you are willing to commit to being in shape you are a long way on the path toward recovery. With energy in the bank, the sky is the limit.

HOW IS IT DONE?

Options for cardiovascular workouts are available for every level of ability and disability. From bed-bound exercises to high-level aerobic workouts, there are many options to work heart and lungs no matter what the level of recovery. A talk with your physical or occupational therapist or athletic trainer can produce suggestions for machines and exercises that build stamina, allow for maximum gains, and keep you safe. Many of the machines that are used for cardio conditioning, including recumbent (reclining) bilateral trainers (see the subheading Cardiovascular Machines in the chapter Recovery Machines, page 169), recumbent stationary bicycles, and upper body exercisers, are appropriate for stroke survivors. There are even treadmills for wheelchairs that build cardiovascular strength. Many of the options are low cost. For instance, portable, combination lower- and upper-body stationary cycles cost about $50. A company called Isokinetics (www.isokineticsinc.com) has five models of pedal exercisers that are appropriate for arm or leg exercise. The cost is between $20 and $78.

Many local hospitals and rehabilitation hospitals have "cardio gyms" for folks rehabilitating from chronic conditions. These gyms are open to stroke survivors and are staffed with knowledgeable therapists who can help direct workouts. These gyms typically require a doctor's prescription. Insurance companies are sometimes willing to pay for memberships to these gyms if your workouts are seen as necessary for recovery and/or overall health.

For stroke survivors who cannot yet walk, **partial weight supported walking** (**PWSW**) equipment can be used at home. For example, both the NeuroGym® Bungee Walker and the Biodex Unweighing System are available for home use (see Recovery Machines, page 169).

WHAT PRECAUTIONS SHOULD BE TAKEN?

Ask your physical or occupational therapist to review the many options available to develop cardiovascular strength. Many of these options can be used within your home. Involving your doctor and rehabilitation professional to guide you toward safe and effective cardiovascular strengthening options is essential.

Recovery Strategies

INTERVENTION SOUP: MIX AND MATCH

Some things are just better together; Wine and cheese, baseball and beer, good friends. One option at a time can work well, but sometimes adding a second (or third, or fourth...) option can magnify and complement both. The same is true of recovery options. These recovery options include:

- Treatment techniques
- Interventions
- Modalities
- Therapies
- Exercises
- Technologies used for recovery
- Any other effort made toward recovery

HOW IS IT DONE?

Mixing and matching (recovery) options is a little like cooking soup. When you cook soup, you taste as you cook. As you add and subtract things to your recovery mix, "taste" the effectiveness of your mix of options.

Adding new options can keep things exciting and, if done correctly, can amplify the efficiency of your recovery routine. The trick is adding a new element and then accurately evaluating if the new element provides a benefit. Finding the correct mix is part science, part art, part intuition, and part experience. There are no rules or flowcharts to direct you through the process of deciding if, what, and when, a set of recovery options works.

Some variables that you need to consider when mixing and matching therapies include:

- *Dosage*. Most people think of dosage as something that relates to drugs, but recovery options have dosages as well. Dosage is simply the "how much" of the option you've chosen. Dosage is defined by:
  — *Amount of time*. This would include the amount of time and the number of times per week you spend doing the option. For instance, if you and your doctor have decided that electrical stimulation helps reduce your spasticity, then the amount of time

that you have the stimulation on would help determine the dosage.

— *Intensity*. Again, using electrical stimulation as the example, the level of stimulation (usually measured in milliamps) would help determine the dosage.

• *Type of stroke.*
 — For example, an option may be safe and effective for someone who had a "block" stroke (ischemic, where the blood vessel was blocked). The same option may not be safe for someone who has had a "bleed" stroke (hemorrhagic, where a blood vessel has burst).

• *Side (left or right side of brain) of damage and if the stroke affected the dominant side.*
 — For example, trying to use **repetitive practice** during writing when it is your nonwriting hand that is affected, would not be helpful to recovery.

• *How long after the stroke it has been.*
 — Some options work well right after the stroke. Other options are best tried once you are in the chronic (after months to 1 year) stage of recovery.

• *The amount of spasticity you have.*
 — If spasticity is strong, it is sometimes wise to focus on options that reduce spasticity before starting other options.

• *The type and number of conditions related to the stroke* (e.g., eyesight problems, loss of feeling, spasticity, aphasia, etc.).

• *The type and number of health issues that are unrelated to the stroke* (e.g., diabetes, heart problems, depression, etc.).

• *Your motivation level.*

• Some options take a tremendous amount of focused effort. You may not be willing to make that effort, sometimes for understandable reasons ("I have grandchildren to take care of; I don't have time!"). Even if an option is something you do not want to consider, that does not mean that your efforts should end. It simply means that different options should be explored.

- *The amount of movement you have.*
  — For instance, options that are effective for someone who has near-perfect movement may not be appropriate for someone who is completely limp on the affected side.

The list of variables continues extensively. There are so many considerations in stroke recovery that it is impossible to develop a perfect system to guide you through the process, and even if there was, new research, technologies, and techniques are developed every day. This makes the situation so fluid that the best advice is to always consider new options and accurately and regularly assess progress.

- *Always include options that challenge you.* No progress comes from simply doing what you can. Recovery comes from continually striving for what you are not yet able to do.
- *Consider technology.* The future of rehabilitation is technology. Why? Because there are 50 million stroke survivors worldwide, and the profit motive is too great for inventors to overlook. Fortunately, this means that inventors spend an enormous amount of money on stroke-recovery research. Keep your eye out for emerging technologies to add to your options.
- *As much as you can, choose options with a direct impact on what you love to do.* The part of your life that you most want to get back is a powerful motivator.
- *Always include aerobic (heart and lung) exercises* into your mix of options.
- *Look for options that do well in clinical research.* See page 183 for easy ways to find out what researchers reject and support. Appendix/ Resources at end of book or Stroke Recovery Research Made Quick And Easy
- *Emphasize options that you can do safely* by yourself, at home.

WHAT PRECAUTIONS SHOULD BE TAKEN?

If you take two or more perfectly safe therapies and add them together they can become dangerous. For instance, imagine if you decide to follow aqua (pool) therapy with treadmill training. The two forms of exercises may work well together, but in the short term, they represent a large increase in the amount of stress on your muscles. If you neglect to take into account the increased fatigue that the aqua therapy adds, these two therapies can be dangerous. For example, imagine getting out of the pool, getting dressed, climbing on the treadmill, and then falling because of fatigued arms and legs.

Keep your doctor informed about changes in your recovery options.

✳   ✳   ✳

LIFESTYLE AS THERAPY

There are not enough hours in a day to accomplish what you need to do, while working the full-time job of recovering from a stroke. However, there are errands, chores, and everyday tasks that can be done in a way that promotes recovery. Sure, daily tasks will take a bit longer, but think of the time and money saved if recovery efforts and everyday chores are combined!

Incorporate recovery efforts into the natural rhythm of your life. For instance, within the boundaries of safety, take the stairs, walk to the store, and use the affected hand to do everything from turning the pages of the newspaper to playing catch with grandchildren. Folding clothes is an excellent way to incorporate **bilateral training** (see The Good Trains the Bad—Bilateral Training, page 93). Accomplishing simple tasks while focusing on the affected extremities will help improve overall coordination, skill, strength, and functional ability. It is important to understand how valuable everyday tasks are to your recovery. Research has three buzzword concepts that form the foundation of all recovery:

- *Repetitive*: doing the movements that you want to relearn over and over
- *Task specific*: having recovery efforts center on specific, real-world tasks
- *Massed practice*: dedicating multiple hours per day to your recovery effort

You can see how using everyday tasks as therapy has the potential to incorporates all three of these concepts.

HOW IS IT DONE?

Clearly, the best way to improve walking after stroke is to walk a lot (see Walking Your Way to Better Walking, page 165). What if you walk to the store, library, or school? For instance, books have to be returned to the library, which is five blocks away. Certainly it would be faster to take the car, but the walk has inherent therapeutic value. Walking is a great exercise and can be naturally incorporated into your lifestyle.

A task such as putting away groceries is a great way to do everything from challenging balance to practicing hand grasp and release. Forgoing the elevator for the stairs challenges you by asking for a large amount of lift at the ankle. Painting helps movements at the wrist, elbow, and shoulder, even if you need to place the brush in your "bad" hand with help from your "good" hand. For someone who loves to paint, painting is an example of a meaningful activity. Research has shown that the more meaningful the activity is to you, the more recovery that activity will promote. Some activities are meaningful to everyone, such as walking, eating, and bathing. Other activities have a special meaning to people with special passions, such as playing a musical instrument, playing golf, or painting.

The trick, of course, is taking the extra time needed to fully incorporate the affected arm and leg into whichever task you choose. Taking extra time for these tasks will also help you stay safe. Rushing will hurt everything from coordination to balance, so take your time for the sake of quality of movement and your own safety.

WHAT PRECAUTIONS SHOULD BE TAKEN?

Stroke survivors should challenge themselves with everyday tasks. However, it would be wise to always question the safety of attempting even the simplest of tasks. For instance, even a walk to the end of the block can be dangerous if you fatigue easily or you're prone to falling. Reaching up to put a cup in a cupboard may help activate grasp and release, challenge balance, and improve coordination, but this same task can be dangerous if you lose your balance. Stroke survivors should be aware of the dangers of pushing themselves into new and challenging tasks, including inherent dangers from loss of balance, falls, spikes in blood pressure, and so forth.

YOUR WORK SCHEDULE

Studies have shown that in hospitals, stroke survivors spend just over an hour per day involved in recovery efforts. In skilled nursing clinics, where many stroke survivors end up after their hospital stay, the situation is not much better. The amount of time paid for by Medicare for all therapies, combined, is just over two hours per day. But in order for the brain to rewire, much more time is needed for recovery of movement. For instance, traditional **constraint-induced therapy**, which is proven to promote recovery, has patients do 6 to 8 hours a day of therapy! Recovery efforts are more effective when they are done many hours a day. The brain rewiring needed to recover can happen during shorts bursts of time, as measured in number of weeks (1-10 weeks), but the number of hours per day should be as high as you can tolerate.

HOW IS IT DONE?

You can tell how much time per day to spend on recovery with a simple test: How much time does it take to get really good at any skill you've ever acquired? Many of the skills and abilities that we've acquired throughout our lives take years of dedicated practice. And we are happy to do it because we are acquiring a new skill. Stroke recovery has the disadvantage of not involving any movement or skill that is new. You are simply relearning what you once knew how to do well. Still, the challenge of recovery can be exhilarating, but only if you are willing to put in the work and the time needed to show results.

The optimal amount of time that should be spent on any given treatment, exercise, or modality is one of the hot topics of stroke-recovery research. Deciding the exact amount of time to spend on recovery efforts can be tricky. It is, however, safe to say that dedicating enough time to recovery can be summarized with the phrase: *recovery is a full-time job*.

Of course, doing 8 hours of work may sound exhausting. Your recovery plan should include options that mix hard physical work with restful work, like mental practice (see Imagine It!, page 78). Always balance between work and rest and between maintaining challenge and safety. Often you will not have to do a particular therapy for a long duration of time, as measured in weeks, months, or years. You might instead have an intense experience with a recovery tool for relatively short bursts (2-3 weeks) of time. Of course, if a recovery option works for longer than that, keep doing it. On the other hand, if a therapy loses its effectiveness or does not work in a relatively short amount of time, then pitch it. Worthwhile therapies tend to show pretty immediate results. Results have to be measured to determine effectiveness. For suggestions on measurements, see Measuring Progress, page 16.

Many stroke survivors are reluctant to put considerable amounts of time into recovery without the guarantee of gains. And there are no guarantees. You may work very hard and recover very little. Efforts toward recovery are a leap of faith. Much of what we do involves leaps of faith, from raising children to getting an education. A full life is full of leaps of faith. Stroke recovery is another leap. Keeping the faith is essential to recovery.

WHAT PRECAUTIONS SHOULD BE TAKEN?

The exact amount of effort toward recovery is a decision to be made by the stroke survivor and his or her doctor. Doctors are experts at determining how much work is safe. A balance should be reached between effectively challenging the stroke survivor without pushing him or her to the point of exhaustion. Overexertion will lead to diminished recovery and, finally, to discouragement and quitting.

✳   ✳   ✳

LIVING RECOVERY

What do you remember from your childhood? Usually it's one of two types of experiences; something good or something bad. Your first kiss and a broken wrist are examples of memories that come back as crystal clear as a photograph. These experiences tend to "hard-wire" into the brain because of their intensity. They have a deep impact that makes you remember the sights, sounds, and emotions of the experience. Intense memories are actually physical in form. They are the connection of particular brain nerve cells firing in a particular order. Think of rehabilitation in much the same way. When the act of recovery becomes as intense an experience as possible, recovery from stroke can shift into high gear.

HOW IS IT DONE?

The more of the whole person, heart and soul, committed to the movement, the more that movement will be remembered. Intensity of emotion and depth of experience can promote recovery by "hard-wiring" the experience. Doctors on the cutting edge of stroke-recovery research talk about patients "driving their nervous system" toward recovery. How can a stroke survivor drive her nervous system, in this case the nerve cells in the brain, toward recovery?

- The effort should be intrinsic, meaningful, and passionate. Think of recovery as a challenging vision quest.
- With each instance of committed effort, the brain is slightly altered toward recovery.
- The effort has to be strong enough, focused enough, and personally powerful enough to drive change.
- Any athlete or musician will tell you the same thing: You have to live it.
- When working toward recovery, effort has to be as intensely experienced as you can make it within the limits of safety.

There are many ways that people use depth of experience to change their lives. The experiences at retreats and camps, for example, can change you in profound ways, in relatively short periods of time. Consider these two experiences:

- Joe plays 2 hours of basketball, every Saturday, for a year. That's a total of 104 hours of total playing time.
- Jim goes to basketball camp for two weeks and plays for 7 hours a day. That's 7 hours a day for 14 days, for total 98 hours of total playing time.

So Joe the "weekend warrior" plays for a total of 104 hours and Jim, the "camper" plays 98 hours. Most researchers now believe that Jim the camper would get better at basketball because he would be much more immersed in the experience than Joe. Jim's camp would make him a better basketball player because of the rich and emotional experience which is, quite literally, imprinted on his brain.

WHAT PRECAUTIONS SHOULD BE TAKEN?

Any time one considers any difficult physical endeavor, whether it's running a marathon or dedicating fully to recovery from stroke, the precautions are the same: Keep your practice within safe boundaries. There is an old Clint Eastwood line, "A man's got to know his limitations." This is true for anyone trying to recover from stroke. It's a recurring theme in this book: intense, strong, serious, and, most importantly, safe. Consult your doctor about any effort in your recovery that you are unsure about.

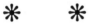

KEEP THE CORE VALUES CLOSE

This book, like any book, can be a reference because it is permanent. Read it, and then put it on the shelf to refer to when you need it. But the fundamental recovery principles should be memorized and more than memorized; they should become an intrinsic part of the recovery process. Keep this book on your shelf. Keep the core values in this book closer.

The basic elements of successful recovery from stroke are remarkably simple. Here is a quick core values cheat sheet of stroke rehabilitation:

HOW IS IT DONE?

- Develop a plan.
- Don't accept that there will be no more significant recovery.
- Continually research new recovery alternatives.
- Incorporate tasks that are meaningful to you into your recovery efforts.
- Use affected "bad" extremities as much as possible.
- Exercise is good.
- Strengthen your muscles.

- Strengthen your cardiovascular system.
- Stretch often.
- Control your weight.
- Treat efforts toward recovery like a full-time job.
- If you can, walk a lot.
- Take every precaution not to fall.
- Within the boundaries of safety, always challenge yourself.
- Measure progress often.
- Fall in love with the process of recovery.

WHAT PRECAUTIONS SHOULD BE TAKEN?

Common sense and your doctor should be your guides.

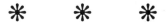

HARD BUT SAFE

Efforts toward recovery should extend you beyond your current ability while remaining safe. This balance is not difficult to achieve, but does require some planning and consultation with your doctor and other health-care providers.

When developing a strategy for recovery from stroke, ask yourself two basic questions:

1. Is it safe?
2. Is it challenging?

If it is safe but not challenging, it will not produce results. If it is challenging but not safe, there is a risk of injury. Pick recovery options that are physically challenging but have little risk.

HOW IS IT DONE?

Some inherently dangerous therapies can be modified to make them safe. An example of this is cardiovascular (heart and lungs) training. You could try to swim, attempt to walk briskly, or ride a bicycle. All of these are healthy for your heart and lungs, but they are all dangerous for some folks who have had a stroke. On the other hand, you can modify any recovery option to be safe. For instance, you can change swimming to aqua therapy (therapy done against the resistance of water). And you can use a stationary recumbent bicycle instead of a regular bicycle. Consider walking. Walking is one of the best, if not the best cardiovascular workouts. If there is a risk of falls or if you are unable to walk, develop a cardiovascular workout that is done in the sitting position. Suggestions for cardio training in the seated position include "ergometers" (stationary cycles for the arms or legs) and recumbent steppers. See page 170 for further examples of machines that help with a cardiovascular workout and that use the legs but do not involve walking. Once you are able to stand, walking can be done with your weight supported or on a treadmill with bars to hold. The worst thing to do, of course, is to assume that walking safely is a lost cause. Giving up on any skill (like walking) may well guarantee more than just losing that skill. It may also provide an opportunity for a downward spiral where lowered expectations lead to less activity, which leads to less strength and stamina, which, in turn, leads to even lower expectations. Workouts designed to increase heart and lung stamina as well as strengthen muscles will help build the foundation needed to walk safely again. There are other "preambulation" techniques that can be used to foster walking, like partial weight supported walking, the NeuroGym® Bungee Walker, and the Biodex Unweighing System.

The "hard but safe" idea is a cornerstone of rehabilitation therapy and rehabilitation research:

- *Hard (challenging)*: All recovery comes from challenge. In many ways, all recovery is "forced." You put yourself in situations where you can barely achieve the goal, and the challenge itself drives recovery. The irony of stroke is that the deficits left by the stroke provide the perfect challenges needed to come back from the stroke. Stroke survivors and well-meaning clinicians often spend much of their effort trying to eliminate the challenge. The saddest situation is when stroke survivors cannot challenge themselves because they don't understand the importance of the challenge. In other cases, survivors are so flaccid (limp) on the affected side that they can't even begin to attempt to meet the challenge. Sometimes stroke survivors, who are asked to move their fingers (or wrist or foot, etc.), deny that they have any movement. A concerned doctor might say, "Humor me, and give it a try," and sure enough, there is movement. Not much movement, but enough to apply **repetitive practice**, rewire the brain, and begin an upward spiral of recovery. Challenge feeds recovery. Recovery feeds on challenge.

- *Safe*: There are two reasons to stress safety:
  1. Injuries are bad; everyone knows this, and everyone knows why. A simple slip and fall can lead to a broken bone, a hospital stay, a pressure sore, and even death.
  2. Injuries stop recovery. The threshold for an injury that stops recovery is much lower than anything that involves a hospital stay. A torn muscle, a sore back, or a bruise can slow or stop recovery efforts.

WHAT PRECAUTIONS SHOULD BE TAKEN?

Inherent in designing an effective rehabilitation program is a commitment to new and challenging areas of physical experience. This is as true with stroke survivors as it is with athletes, musicians, dancers, and other individuals who use their bodies to express themselves, pursue their passions, and make their living. The trick for survivors is to make the rehabilitation efforts both challenging and effective while remaining safe. Consulting your doctor and involving physical, occupational, and other health-care providers will go a long way in maintaining the safety-challenge dynamic.

✳ ✳ ✳

EAT TO RECOVER

Diet has huge implications on so many levels for everyone. From its effect on diseases like diabetes and vascular disease to the effect on the immune system and mental acuity, what you eat has a huge impact on your quality of life. The impact of diet on stroke survivors is even larger than on the general population because diet can affect many aspects of stroke recovery including energy levels, physical performance, mood, cardiovascular health (stroke is a cardiovascular disease), and muscle strength. Maintaining optimal weight helps to make movement easier. The opposite is true as well; increases in weight gain make recovery harder because weight gained is weight that has to be lifted during movement. Stroke survivors tend to cascade toward weight gain. The heavier a stroke survivor is over his or her optimum weight, the more difficult the path to physical recovery. In some folks, stroke initiates a downward spiral that might look like this:

Stroke—>

Survivor is less active—>

Survivor gains weight—>

Added weight promotes inactivity—>

The survivor gains more weight—>

And so on—>

Downward pattern of weight gain in stroke survivors.

HOW IS IT DONE?

So, what exactly is the correct diet for someone rehabbing from stroke? Lots of useful information in libraries, on the web, and with health professionals will provide all the specific diet suggestions you'll ever need. Here are a few basic dietary guidelines for anyone trying to improve physical performance:

- *Try to remain within your optimum weight.* It's a lot easier to lift your arm if it weighs 20 pounds than if it weighs 30 pounds. Your doctor can tell you your optimum weight. Weight beyond your optimum makes training after stroke difficult because extra weight is weight that has to be lifted, shifted, and held whenever you move. Also, unnecessary fat needs to be vascularized (blood vessels need to be manufactured by your body to feed the extra cells). This extra vascularization makes the heart have to work that much harder to pump that much more blood to these new vessels.
- *Choose quality carbohydrates.* Carbohydrates can be bad (processed)

or good (unprocessed). Carbohydrates, after being digested, are deposited in the blood stream as sugar.

— Processed (also known as refined or simple) carbohydrates like white rice, potato chips, pretzels, white bread, white sugar, candy, sodas, etc., are digested and absorbed into the blood quickly. Because this process happens rapidly, there is a spike in blood sugar. The quick release of sugars puts stress on the insulin delivery system that maintains optimum sugar balance. Enough of these roller coaster rides of sugar levels and type 2 diabetes can develop. Also, spikes in sugar lead to a reaction in the body, which quickly stores the blood sugar. This process leaves you feeling hungry again.

— Unprocessed (also known as unrefined or complex) carbohydrates like whole grain bread, brown rice, and whole fruits (apples, oranges, etc.) provide a much more gradual digestion of the carbohydrate, resulting in a much more gradual release of sugar. The slower the release of sugar, the better, because a gradual release can be better absorbed, stored, and used by the body.

• *Stay away from hydrogenated and partially hydrogenated fats.* Hydrogenated fats are oils that are heated and once they cool, stay solid at room temperature. Partially hydrogenated fats are oils that are heated so they are somewhere between solid and liquid at room temperature. Hydrogenated and partially hydrogenated oils are found in fried foods and are ingredients in pastries, chips, cookies, crackers, muffins, donuts, candy, and much of fast food. These bad fats are written in the ingredients list on a food package as hydrogenated vegetable oil, partially hydrogenated vegetable oil, or shortening. The flipside to the oil equation is increasing good fats in your diet. Good fats include extra virgin olive oil, fish oil, cod-liver oil, nut oil, flaxseed oil, and canola oil. Good fats will actually lower the level of bad fats. These good fats can have health-boosting qualities. High levels of good fats before a stroke decrease memory loss and disability after a stroke.

• *Eat a lot of fresh fruits and vegetables.* Fruits and vegetables have important vitamins, minerals, and amino acids (the building blocks of proteins). Fruits and veggies should be eaten in a state that is as unprocessed as possible. Processed means cooked and/or combined with other ingredients. For instance, simply slicing a fruit or vegetable will reduce the amount of vitamins and minerals it has because some of the nutrient-rich juice is lost. Fruits and vegetables that are unprocessed and fresh will provide the greatest nutritional value. Fruits and vegetables help satiate your hunger, which keeps you from eating less healthy foods.

One habit that is essential to a healthy diet is simply reading the ingredients of what it is you eat. Reading the ingredients will lead to simple but profound questions like:

- "What is that ingredient?"
- "Why is that chemical in this food?"
- "How does this food compare to its whole (unprocessed) version?"

These questions inevitably lead to better dietary choices because they provide information about what you are eating, and help you to question why you eat what you do.

Buildup in the walls of arteries, the blood vessels that carry blood from the heart to all the cells in the body, is the cause of many strokes. This buildup is called plaque. High levels of a chemical called homocysteine can cause plaque buildup. People who have had a stroke have a tendency toward high blood levels of homocysteine. This may be a problem that is easily solved. Ask your doctor about the use of vitamin B12 to reduce levels of homocysteine. It is worth noting that high levels of homocysteine also increase your chance of disability after stroke.

Stroke can affect your ability to taste. Stroke can make foods taste weird, bad, or it can reduce your ability to taste at all. There is even a word for this change in the ability to taste after brain injury: *dysgeusia*. There may be a tendency to overcome the lack of taste by adding taste enhancers like salt, extra sauces and spices, or frying foods. Be prudent and healthy with your choices as you attempt to make food palatable.

WHAT PRECAUTIONS SHOULD BE TAKEN?

Inform your doctor about any major changes in your diet, even if they are considered healthy. For instance, switching to a vegetarian diet may be considered healthy but may not be appropriate for you at this time.

✳   ✳   ✳

MAKE HOME MOVIES

Videotaping your recovery efforts can provide all sorts of information about your recovery. Researchers use all sorts of sophisticated and expensive tests to determine if a therapy is working. From brain imaging to computers that measure joint angles, researchers attempt to get the most accurate data possible. But at the end of the day, some of the most convincing information comes from simple videotape. Why is video so important? Because we humans are visual beings, and we believe what we see.

You can use the information that video provides to evaluate many different aspects of your recovery. Some of the questions to think about when reviewing your videotapes include:

- Is movement quality improving?
- Are movements performed faster but with the same or better coordination?
- Is walking more fluid and coordinated?
- Is there a reduction of tremor (shaking)?
- Is targeting (ability to move a body part into a space at which you are aiming) better?
- Are movements more symmetrical?
- Is a given task completed with more coordination and finesse?
- Are tasks attempted performed better than before?
- Do any movements look incorrect for any reason?
- Do you seem to be in any danger when you move? Do you see that you are at risk for falling?

In the short term, video can provide valuable feedback about body position, timing, duration, and quality of movement, among many other aspects of recovery. First, you take a video of yourself performing a task, and then immediately watch the tape. As you view the tape, make a mental note on how you can improve in the future. Athletes use videotaping in this way all the time. A golfer will take a video of his swing and then watch the video and critique his swing. This feedback allows you to view the task almost immediately but, unlike viewing the task in a mirror, you can fully and objectively concentrate on the quality of movement. In this way, videotaping can provide short-term feedback.

Video can provide long-term feedback as well. Recovery tends to be seamless and gradual. It is difficult for you to objectively view progress unless there is a way to review where you started. Once you see that you've improved, you'll be motivated to improve even more. Video delivers "Ah-ha!" moments as you realize that movements or tasks can now be accomplished that, just a few days (or weeks or months) ago, were impossible.

Audio recordings can be made to evaluate speech. Audio recordings may have advantages over video recordings of speech because the wide range of oral maneuvers that stroke survivors use to formulate words often look uncoordinated but produce the best and most understandable speech. Audiotape will help you focus on the quality of your speech, rather than what it looks like. On the other hand, there may be times when you want to see the way your mouth is moving. There are two kinds of problems with speech that may result after stroke: aphasia and dysarthria. **Aphasia** is damage to the word-processing part of the brain. **Dysarthria** is a problem with the part of the brain that controls movement at the mouth. Someone with dysarthria may benefit from seeing how his or her mouth, lips, and tongue are moving on a video.

HOW IS IT DONE?

All you need is a video camera. Inexpensive and pocket-sized digital cameras can go wherever you go. Most computers can be rigged with an inexpensive video camera, which puts the video right on your computer. From there you can keep the various videos organized and categorized on the computer. Digital video from your portable camera can be uploaded and organized onto your home computer as well.

It may be helpful to take video from several different angles (front, side, back, etc.). Once a video is made, note where and when it was made. Use the same or similar environments, footwear, objects, and so forth, to make future comparisons more accurate. Keep the movements or tasks consistent through all your videos. This will help you compare apples to apples. Focus on quality of movement more than speed, unless speed is essential to the task. Researchers will often test at two speeds: fast and self-selected (the speed at which you are most comfortable for that movement). When researchers and therapists test the movement of stroke survivors, they try to capture the best movement possible. They want the stroke survivor to try to perform the task as if he or she never had a stroke. When you are videotaping, it may help to first take a video of someone who has not had a stroke. Have them perform the same movement in an "ideal" way. Their movement can be analyzed with respect to your movement, and revealing comparisons can be made.

WHAT PRECAUTIONS SHOULD BE TAKEN?

Do not compromise safety when videotaping. Because you may have to be the subject as well as the photographer, there may be wires, stands, or other equipment that can interfere with safe walking.

✳ ✳ ✳

DON'T NEGLECT THE "GOOD" SIDE

"The squeaky wheel gets the grease." This is true with stroke survivors who often put much of their effort into training the "squeaky" limbs on the affected side. There are a lot of understandable reasons to work on the "bad" side. But there are also good reasons to work with the unaffected side of the body.

HOW IS IT DONE?

Here is an outline of reasons to work the "good" side:

- *Research has shown that stroke affects both sides of the brain and body.* Researchers really don't use the term "unaffected side," they use the term "less affected side." The fact is that both sides are affected by the stroke and can benefit from exercise and coordination training.
- *During parts of the recovery process the "good" side is going to accept more of the responsibility of everyday life.* From dressing to driving, more is going to be asked of the "good" side. Since this side has a greater role, it needs more strength, flexibility, and coordination. For folks whose stroke affects their dominant side (e.g., right side

is affected for someone who is right-handed) new responsibilities are accepted by the nondominant (left) extremity. Some of the new skills will involve fine-dexterity activities like writing and grooming. For this reason, just to continue the activities of daily life, the stroke survivor needs to work on coordination of the less affected side.

- *The "good" side can be used to exercise in ways that the affected side cannot (in the short term).* For example, at some points in recovery, a cardiovascular workout may only be able to be accomplished by the less affected side because the "bad" side has a limited ability to move. But there is still cardiovascular benefit from letting the "good" side do all the work. This is not an invitation to concentrate recovery efforts *only* on the unaffected side. Rather, "working with what you've got" provides a short-term strategy for doing all sorts of strengthening and cardiovascular training at any point during recovery.

- *When both sides are worked together, the affected side is going to fatigue much faster.* Once the "bad" side is too fatigued to work and needs time to rest, recovery efforts can continue by working with the less affected side.

Recovery from stroke often sets survivors on a course to a healthier overall lifestyle. For some people, it fosters an increased attention to health issues. For others, it provides a renewed focus on how their bodies move. This renewed focus on health will lead to working with your body—the whole body—which provides benefits to your health and recovery. Overall health and stroke recovery are intertwined and cannot be separated. Each depends on the other. Using the "good" side to promote overall health will also help recovery.

WHAT PRECAUTIONS SHOULD BE TAKEN?

Lower-extremity exercises done by the unaffected side may place extra strain on the affected leg and foot, leading to falls and resultant injury. Keep this in mind when performing any exercises that challenges balance while standing.

Working hard with the "good" side will challenge the heart and lungs in a way that would otherwise be limited. Because working the unaffected side will encourage an increased intensity of exercises, you should inform your doctor of the intensity increase.

✻   ✻   ✻

GUIDE YOUR DOCTOR

While reading this book you may have found one recurring theme: "Push the issue." In all areas of stroke recovery you should work to achieve, and expect, the most recovery possible. Recovery is best served when you and your caretakers always "push the issue."

Doctors, nurses, and therapists are used to the lowered expectations of the typical stroke survivor. They may assume that you have similar expectations. Stroke survivors can sometimes influence clinicians toward lowered expectations. Clinicians then use what they've learned to influence other stroke survivors. Each influences the other. The bottom line is: Your doctor may not realize that you want to get better. Many doctors still believe that little or no recovery occurs after the "subacute" period (from 3-9 months after stroke). If your plan is to achieve as much recovery as possible, it is going to be unusual and unexpected. It is up to you to let your doctor know that you want to take your recovery as far as it will go, and that you want them on your recovery team. Doctors will be motivated to push the issue if you are motivated; both of your ambitions will feed off each other. Consider your relationship with your doctor as a partnership dedicated to your recovery.

HOW IS IT DONE?

When you talk to your doctor about your recovery from stroke, keep it simple. Talk to your doctor about specific problems, issues, and thoughts. For instance, don't say something general like, "I want to move better." Instead, focus on more specific problems relating to movement deficits.

For example, spasticity will often cause the hand to be postured in a tight fist. This will make the hand difficult to open and difficult to clean. Also, the nails become difficult to trim. Because of the strength of the fist, the nails begin to cut into the hand. This specific problem requires specific attention. In this case, you would tell your doctor that your nails are cutting into your hand, and that you want to be able to open the hand. The doctor then can provide a specific treatment that will target that specific problem.

As you discuss your recovery with your doctor, keep the following two goals in mind:

- *Convince your doctor that you are going to "push the issue."* You have made the decision to go forward no matter what the naysayers claim and despite what your body is (sometimes) telling you. Let your doctor know that you need him to help you in this vision quest.
- *Talk to your doctor about the effectiveness and safety of the next series of treatment* options in your plan. That is, you have to let him know what the short-term plan is. Focusing on the short-term portion of your plan will help retain your doctor's focus and enthusiasm.

Here are suggestions when visiting with your doctor:

- Bring a written list of questions.
- Bring a written list of goals that you want to achieve.
- Bring an advocate (friend, family member, or caregiver) with you. Discuss with your advocate what you want to know and why you want to know it before the appointment, so if you forget a question, they can chime in.
- Bring a list of prescription medications, over-the-counter medications, and supplements you are taking. Discuss how your medications might be affecting your recovery.
- Be prepared to take notes. Bring a pencil and paper or a tape recorder.
- Suggest that your doctor write a script (prescription) for occupational, physical, and speech therapy, if therapy is needed to achieve the next step in your recovery.
- Get feedback from the doctor on treatment options that you've researched and are thinking of implementing.

Keep two things in mind when choosing doctors:

1. *Your primary doctor may not be knowledgeable about the cutting-edge recovery options* that you will need, from time to time, to continue

progressing toward recovery. A physiatrist (see A Doctor Made for Stroke Survivors, page 10) is a doctor who specializes in rehabilitation. Consider having your primary doctor refer you to a physiatrist. Physiatrists will be knowledgeable about the use of cutting-edge recovery options. They will also have specialized tools that will help you during your recovery quest.

2. *Some doctors are not aggressive.* If the doctor you choose does not understand your ambitious plan, get another doctor. This is especially true for the specialists (neurologists and physiatrists) who will need to be on-board your plan for you to recover.

WHAT PRECAUTIONS SHOULD BE TAKEN?

Push the issue!

Spasticity Control and Elimination

SPASTICITY—THE BEAST UNMASKED

WHAT IS IT?

Spasticity is a disorder that is rarely fully explained to stroke patients. Clinicians tend to describe spasticity in terms of its effect on limbs. For instance they may say, "The stroke causes the hand to be tight." Or they may say, "Your muscles are tightening because of the damage caused to your brain by the stroke." These explanations of spasticity are incomplete. You need the whole story. Without an understanding of the cause of spasticity there is little chance of reducing spasticity. Spasticity reduction, like most of stroke recovery, comes from the inside out. Only the stroke survivor can reduce her spasticity. Like so many other aspects of stroke recovery the stroke survivor needs to be in the "driver's seat" on the road toward recovery. *Information*, if you follow the metaphor, is the roadmap.

HOW IS IT DONE?

How can spasticity be reduced or eliminated in a way that does not involve drugs or surgery? The only way to silence spasticity is to restore control of the spastic muscles to the brain. Using the **neuroplastic** process is the only way to restore control of the muscles. You have to understand what spasticity is in order to use the neuroplastic process to combat it.

Here is an explanation of spasticity that is scientifically correct and, hopefully, easy to understand:

How muscles work:
- Your muscles send constant messages to the brain about the amount of tension the muscle is feeling. If muscles have too much tension they will tear, so the brain and muscles are in a constant dance to make sure that the muscle is helping you move and is also safe from tearing.

How the brain works before stroke:
- Your brain tells your muscles when to contract (tighten to help you move).
- Your brain also tells your muscles *when to relax.*

How the brain works after stroke:
- Stroke kills part of the brain responsible for movement of muscles.
- After stroke, the brain no longer "hears" the affected muscles.
- The brain no longer tells affected muscle when to contract or when to relax.

But there is another player in this game. If your brain is not fully able to control your muscles, what makes them tight? Are the muscles acting alone? Or is something telling them to tighten?

How the spinal cord causes spasticity:
- Muscles constantly send signals to the spinal cord, and the spinal cord sends those signals up to the brain.
- After stroke, the brain is no longer capable of listening to the signals the muscles send out.
- Muscles do not like to be stretched too much. They tear easily.
- Impulses from the spinal cord protect muscles by keeping them short (contracted).

The impulse that the spinal cord sends out to protect muscles is similar to the stretch reflex caused by a reflex hammer that a doctor uses to hit you right below the kneecap, causing your knee to extend. The knee extends whether you want it to or not. The movement of the leg kicking forward is called a *stretch reflex*. The stretch reflex exists to instantly protect the muscle from tearing by shortening the muscles on the front upper part of your leg. This causes the knee to extend. Imagine if the doctor hit the knee over and over and never stopped. Spasticity can be viewed as an ongoing repetition of reflexes.

What spasticity does:
- The spinal cord tells the muscles to remain contracted (shortened). This command *is* spasticity.
- In a matter of weeks, spasticity will permanently shorten muscles.
- The shortened muscle perceives any lengthening as a threat of tearing.
- The muscle sends out an increased amount of *"Help! I'm tearing!"* messages to the brain and spinal cord.
- The spinal cord continues to send signals to the muscle to tighten.

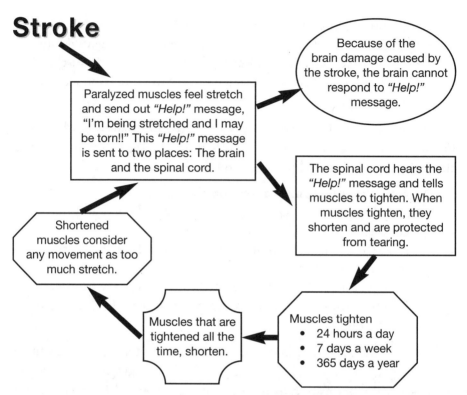

A representation of the process of spasticity in the stroke survivor.

And around and around it goes: the muscle keeps saying "Help!" and the spinal cord says "Contract!" This process makes the muscle tighten even more, causing more "Help!" signals from the muscle. This process is ongoing and continues even during sleep.

WHAT PRECAUTIONS SHOULD BE TAKEN?

None.

✱   ✱   ✱

NEUROPLASTIC BEATS SPASTIC

After a stroke, the brain can no longer protect the muscle from being over-stretched and torn. So the spinal cord takes over and tells the muscles to stay tight, which protects them from being torn. Spasticity is a protection mechanism. The problem, of course, is that tight muscles make it difficult to move.

No drugs, therapies, or modalities will permanently eliminate spasticity. There is hope, however. Hiding in plain sight, the answer to the riddle of spasticity may simply be to exercise the spastic muscles. At the bottom of this idea is our old friend, **neuroplasticity**. Recovery efforts that rewire the brain can be used so that more brain "real estate" is dedicated to the spastic muscles. As the brain regains control, spasticity is no longer necessary. Muscle tightness will become less intense which will, in turn, provide more control of movement.

The following is a partial list of recovery options that has been used to drive brain-rewiring.

- Repetitive practice
- Mental practice
- Constraint-induced therapy
- Functional electrical stimulation orthotics
- Robotics
- Bilateral training
- Virtual reality

HOW IS IT DONE?

The downward spiral after stroke

Stroke ⟹ Part of brain that controls muscles is damaged ⟹ Brain cannot control, nor protect, muscles ⟹ Spinal cord protects muscles by making them tight ⟹ Muscles permanently shorten ⟹ Tight, shortened muscles make movement difficult.

The upward spiral after stroke

Stretching retains muscle length and repetitive practice rewires the brain ⟹ Brain regains responsibility of muscle control ⟹ Spinal cord gives control of muscles to brain ⟹ Spasticity declines or is eliminated ⟹ Movement is made more normal.

The only way to permanently reduce or eliminate spasticity is by rewiring the brain to regain control over muscles. The same recovery options that promote brain rewiring will reduce spasticity as well. Increased movement and reduced spasticity are two sides of the same coin.

- As spasticity decreases, the ability to move improves.
- The ability to move better chips away at spasticity.

Animal research studies have found that immobilizing a limb will shrink the number of brain cells dedicated to the muscles that move the limb. This is exactly what happens to stroke survivors with spasticity. Their muscles are immobilized by spasticity. If the spastic muscles resume movement, the portion of the brain representing those muscles will get larger. As more brain power goes into those muscles, spasticity will subside.

Treatments that **physiatrists** and neurologists use can help you to rewire your brain to regain control over spastic muscles. These doctors have specialized training in treatments that reduce spasticity. Some drugs and other treatments provide temporary relief from spasticity. The temporary relief can allow for easier movement. Treatments used to reduce spasticity may help create an opportunity for the hard work of rewiring your brain.

Drugs used to reduce spasticity fall into two groups:

- Given locally (injected directly into the spastic muscles) or administered into the fluid surrounding the spinal cord. These drugs affect only specific muscles.
- Taken orally. These drugs will affect all the muscles in your body.

These drugs can reduce spasticity, which can:

- Improve movement
- Increase the potential of recovery
- Curb potential bone and joint problems
- Reduce pain
- Increase strength
- Reduce the risk of **contracture**
- Set the stage for neuroplastic change

Ask your doctor about these options. Remember though, these medications will not address the underlying cause of spasticity (lack of control by the brain over muscles). No drug will replace the hard work needed to rewire your brain. The drugs and other treatments that temporarily reduce spasticity provide a window of opportunity for you to do the hard work of rewiring the brain.

The hard work comes in the form of:

- **Constraint-induced therapy**
- The use of **repetitive, task-specific massed practice**
- Some electrical stimulation treatments
- Some forms of **bilateral training**
- **Mental practice**

This list will grow with emerging research, so continue to explore the research and ask lots of questions.

WHAT PRECAUTIONS SHOULD BE TAKEN?

Consultation with your doctors, therapists, and other health professionals will help direct your therapy so that spasticity reduction is achieved with a minimum of waste and a maximum of treatment effect.

You and your doctor may decide to use spasticity medications for reasons other than offering a window of opportunity for neuroplastic change. There may be other very good reasons for oral and other forms of spasticity medications. Reasons for continued use of systemic spasticity medications may include better mobility, less pain, better movement, etc.

*   *   *

SPASTICITY—JEKYLL AND HYDE?

WHAT IS IT?

In some ways spasticity can be of temporary benefit as you move away from the "flaccid phase" of recovery.

Immediately after their stroke, some survivors are flaccid (limp) on the affected side. Nothing on the affected side can be moved under the survivor's own power. This is a scary time for survivors and their families. It is a cruel joke that stroke survivors are at their worst right after their stroke, when they are least able to understand and react to what has happened to them. Research shows only limited recovery for stroke survivors who remain flaccid for a year after their stroke. But some stroke survivors, who think they are flaccid, are actually not. Part of the problem is the words that are used to describe problems with movement. The word paralyzed is often used by folks to actually mean "hemiparetic." **Hemiparetic** means weakness on one side of the body. The only stroke survivors who are truly paralyzed are folks who are flaccid on the affected side. Flaccid paralysis after stroke is rare. Most stroke survivors fall into a broad category of "hemiparetic." You may think this is a distinction without a difference. But small amounts of movement can be used as a jumping-off point for much larger and more coordinated movement. So there is a huge difference between "no movement" and "small amounts of movement." Someone who is flaccid after a year has a poor prognosis for return of movement. Someone who has small amounts of movement has retained the brain-muscle connection, and growing that connection means greater movement. Growing that connection *is* neuroplasticity.

The **Brunnstrom** stages reveal that, as people recover from stroke, they go from a period of being flaccid and emerge into a period in which they are spastic. Having spasticity emerge is seen as a period of hope because muscles are finally able to contract. With the emergence of spasticity often small amounts of **synergistic movement** occur.

Brunnstrom's stages state that after the flaccid period comes the emergence of spasticity. Can spasticity be viewed in some sort of positive light? The fact is that there are bad *and* good aspects to spasticity.

HOW IS IT DONE?

Spasticity is bad because it:

- Shortens muscles and other **soft tissue**, which can lead to permanent shortening (**contracture**)
- Positions joints abnormally, which makes limbs less functional
- Interferes with normal activities
- May cause pain
- May cause insomnia
- May cause deformities

- May cause poor weight gain (permanently contracted muscles burn a lot of calories)
- May cause pressure sores

Spasticity is good because:

- It is useful protection in cases of "unilateral neglect" (when the stroke survivor is less aware or completely unaware of the affected side). For instance, in the arm and hand, spasticity will pull the limb across the body. This may be more desirable than the flaccid state, in which the limb is flopping around and fingers and arm are at risk for injury.
- It may build bone strength (using **Wolf's law**), reducing the risk of osteoporosis.
- It can be used to substitute for strength, allowing standing, walking, and gripping.
- It sometimes makes transfers (e.g., going from sitting to standing) easier.
- It may improve circulation, preventing blood clots and swelling.
- It maintains muscle bulk.

WHAT PRECAUTIONS SHOULD BE TAKEN?

The emergence of spasticity can be seen as a positive sign in the overall arc of recovery. But once spasticity has been established, the next stage of recovery requires the reduction and eventual elimination of spasticity. The **Brunnstrom** stages dictate that once spasticity appears, the next step in recovery requires the elimination of spasticity. As is true with much of stroke recovery: one job is done, while another begins.

✳   ✳   ✳

GIVE SPASTICITY THE ONE-TWO PUNCH

Health-care workers and stroke survivors sometimes make the mistake of thinking that spasticity in the arm is an arm problem or that spasticity in the leg is a leg problem. One thing is clear: Spasticity is a brain problem. Spasticity is a symptom of the brain damage caused by stroke. Spasticity is a protection mechanism that keeps muscles from being torn. The brain is no longer doing its job, so the spinal cord takes over the job of protecting muscles, joints, and other soft tissue (i.e., nerves, blood vessels, and the muscles themselves). The spinal cord sends out one message, over and over: Muscles, protect yourself! *Tighten!*

Many researchers believe that if enough of the right kind of **neuroplasticity** (brain rewiring) can occur, spasticity will be reduced. But there is a problem. For the neuroplastic process to start, you need the ability to initiate movements. But if spasticity is too strong, then movement becomes impossible. If neuroplasticity needs some movement, but the stroke survivor's limbs and fingers don't move because of spasticity, how do you jump start the process? For some stroke survivors there may be a way.

The drug that can target the specific muscles that are spastic is called Botox® (botulinum toxin type A). Botox® is a brand name for botulinum toxin. Usually physiatrists or neurologists administer Botox®.

Botox® has gotten most of its press because folks use it to get rid of wrinkles. And the way it eliminates wrinkles is important in understanding how it works on spastic muscles. Lines in your face are created and accentuated by the muscles that move your face around during frowning, squinting, and raising the forehead. A doctor can inject Botox®, which paralyzes these muscles and relaxes the muscle's pull on your face, allowing for fewer wrinkles. Botox® works on spastic muscles in the same way: It relaxes spastic muscles.

If you hear the word "botulism" and immediately think of the food poisoning that makes people ill from eating food that has gone bad, you are right. Botox® is made from the same bacteria that causes botulism. That bacteria, called *Clostridium botulinum*, gives off a substance that can paralyze muscles. This substance is harvested from the bacteria to make Botox®. Botox® does not contain the actual bacteria that causes botulism and does not give patients botulism. Botox® decreases the release of acetylcholine, which is a chemical that allows a nerve signal to reach the muscles. In this way, it blocks nerve impulses, like those that cause spasticity.

The combination of Botox® and exercise techniques used to initiate movement can be effective in improving movement and permanently reducing spasticity. Botox® is injected into tight muscles, and those muscles then relax enough to unmask available movement. The idea is to allow for **recovery options that promote brain rewiring** using movement that was impossible to achieve prior to the Botox® treatment. Each treatment with Botox® in spastic muscles usually relaxes the treated muscles for about 3 months. This treatment provides a window of opportunity to increase active (self-propelled) movement. However, Botox® can be administered more than once, so multiple opportunities to increase movement exist.

HOW IS IT DONE?

There is a combination of treatments that, when used properly together, can jump start the process of spasticity reduction and encourage movement. This combination of treatments has three parts:

1. Botox® is injected directly into spastic muscles.
2. (*This step may or may not be necessary*) Electrical stimulation (e-stim) is used to help develop your ability to begin to move, even a little bit. The type of e-stim comes in one or more of three forms:
   - Cyclic e-stim
   - Electromyography (EMG)-based biofeedback e-stim
   - E-stim functional orthotics
3. Options that promote brain rewiring are used.

Example A

Robert cannot lift his affected foot because there is a lot of spasticity in the muscles that force the foot down (the calf muscles). He goes to his doctor. His doctor refers Robert to a physiatrist.

- The physiatrist uses Botox® to relax the calf muscles.
- Once the spastic muscles are relaxed, Robert works hard to lift the foot. He also does a lot of stretching of the calf muscles. His relaxed muscles allow him to stretch more than he has been able to since his stroke. But Robert continues to have trouble lifting his foot, even a little, on his own.
- Robert's physical therapist suggests cyclic (on, off, repeating) **electrical stimulation** on the muscles that lift the foot. Progress is slow, and since Botox® only lasts a few months, Robert suggests to his therapist that he try something he has read about: **electromyogra-**

phy (EMG)-based electrical stimulation.
- The combination of Botox® and the electrical stimulation works. Robert can lift his foot a little bit.
- Robert uses repetitive practice to build muscle and rewire his brain neuroplastically.

Example B

Kathy's hand is always flexed at the wrist and fingers. Spasticity is forcing her hand into a permanent fist, forcing the fingernails into the flesh of the palm. This causes cuts in Kathy's palm and makes her hand difficult to clean. Kathy goes to a neurologist.

- Botox® is used to relax the muscles that are causing the wrist and fingers to bunch up. These muscles are located in the palm side of the forearm.
- Exercises are prescribed by an occupational therapist to stretch the muscles that were tight (the same muscles that got the Botox® treatment) and strengthen the muscles that open the fingers and lift the wrist.
- Despite a lot of effort with the occupational therapist and at home, Kathy can only open her fingers a small amount.
- Kathy's therapist suggests she use an e-stim orthotic on her arm. The orthotic had been tried before with Kathy, but the e-stim was not strong enough to open her hand. But now the Botox® relaxes the hand enough for the e-stim orthotic to work.
- The combination of e-stim and practice of grasp and release allows Kathy to begin to open her hand on her own. Kathy notices that her "new" ability to pick up objects has helped not only her hand, but her elbow and shoulder as well.

Some doctors inject Botox®, but do not use any sort of intervention to build on the opportunity provided by the Botox®. This is a mistake. Botox® does not permanently eliminate spasticity. Instead, it creates opportunities for spasticity to be permanently reduced. After treatment with Botox® there should be some intervention to take advantage of the window of opportunity the drug presents.

Here is a partial list of therapies that may be effective in conjunction with Botox®:

- Virtual reality
- **Repetitive practice**
- **Modified** and classic **constraint-induced therapy** (**mCIT, CIT**)
- Cyclic electrical stimulation
- Electromyography-based electrical stimulation with **biofeedback** (e.g., Mentamove, Neuromove™)
- Stretching programs aimed at the muscles treated
- Traditional occupational and physical therapy (which may include any or all of the therapies in this list)

WHAT PRECAUTIONS SHOULD BE TAKEN?

Doctors, usually physiatrists or neurologists, administer this drug. A doctor will decide if you are an appropriate candidate for Botox® treatment. After Botox® is administered, adjunctive therapy can help foster the muscle relaxation that this treatment provides. Recovery options that involve electrical stimulation have contraindications and precautions. Discuss these with your medical doctor.

Motivation: Recovery Fuel

MEETING THE CHALLENGE OF RECOVERY

Here is an actual conversation I had with a stroke survivor:

HER: OK Pete, you've been involved in stroke-recovery re-
　　search for a long time. What do you have that will
　　help me recover my hand and help my walking?
ME: I have good news and bad news. The good news is that
　　I have a plan that will help you get the most recovery
　　possible.
HER: Great! I was hoping you'd say that!
ME: The bad news is that you'll probably work harder than
　　you've ever worked in your life.
HER: Oh. I was hoping you could come up with something
　　where I didn't have to work hard.

There the conversation ended. She was unconvinced, and something I already knew was confirmed. The elephant in the room is that some stroke survivors don't want to work hard toward recovery. At least this survivor was honest.

Is it possible to maintain motivation, when the going gets (*really*) tough? This is no idle question. Although many claim to be willing to change their lives in profound ways, if the stakes are high enough, more often than not people choose not to change. Consider the stroke survivor who has never been in good physical shape, has never been an athlete, and has never trained hard for physical gains. How is he going to magically transform into a "recovery machine?" How is he going to physically work harder than ever before?

Here are some thoughts about motivation:

- Maintaining motivation during the rigors of recovery is a discipline unto itself.
- It could not be simpler: People who stay motivated make progress.
- Motivation is essential to recovery, and if motivation is consistently maintained, it can drive recovery.
- Motivation is often the factor that has the most influence on recovery.
- Motivation is the core of recovery.

- Recovery from stroke is full of periods of incredible progress as well as disappointing lulls. Overcoming the slow periods and remaining focused is essential to the process of recovery.

People are motivated by a variety of different things. Here are a few quotes from stroke survivors regarding motivation:

- "I need to be independent. I don't want to rely on my family."
- "I have to get my hand and arm back. My weak arm has stopped me from things I love to do with my friends."
- "I want to be able to take care of my children (or grandchildren or great-grandchildren)."
- "I can't function with the constant fear of falling. I have to improve my balance and strengthen my legs."
- "I see my recovery as an adventure. I want to know how far I can go."
- "I don't want to walk funny. It's bad for business."

If you are willing to work hard, maybe harder than you've ever worked, you have the best chance of the highest possible level of recovery. Some survivors feel that the challenge of recovery is one of the defining moments in their lives. Accepting the challenges of recovery can make the difference between simply reclaiming something lost and embarking on a new adventure toward uncharted personal growth.

HOW IS IT DONE?

Motivation is tied to your personal aspirations, ambitions, and dreams. What motivates you toward recovery also depends on what you are unwilling to surrender. These two (what you want to do and what you want back) are powerful internal motivators. But if you do need inspiration from the outside, there are plenty of resources for that. Motivational stories can be found on the Internet, in books, movies, plays, and within one's faith. Books and movies can offer suggestions, and they can provide an opportunity to "experience" someone else making mistakes and finding solutions. In a word, these stories can *inspire*. The books and movies you choose do not have to be stroke specific. They can be stories about athletes, mountain climbers, war heroes, or anyone's story of survival and triumph.

Here are some other ideas for remaining motivated:

- *Recovery takes positive reinforcement.* Celebrate the small successes.
- *Turn recovery into a competition.* Successful athletes always compete against themselves.
- *Make recovery a social activity.* Your success can be fostered with the help of others, even if they are not stroke survivors.
- *Look for intensity of experience during recovery.* The intensity of the experience will help ingrain what is being learned.
- *Fall in love with the process of recovery.*
- *Have a recovery plan that includes measurable goals.* Success should be measured.
- *Make recovery efforts a part of your everyday schedule.*

The challenge of recovery is at once tenuous, difficult, fraught with frustration, and full of fits and starts. But like a four-wheel-drive vehicle through banks of snow, hard work can compensate for much of the difficult terrain. Researchers are just beginning to unravel the riddle of recovery. The secret seems to be obvious: Recovery takes a tremendous amount of hard and sometimes frustrating work. Hard work drives cardiovascular and muscular strengthening. Hard work goes into planning and stroke-recovery research. And hard work is what will power through plateaus and forge the neuroplastic process.

WHAT PRECAUTIONS SHOULD BE TAKEN?

The often-uncharted territory involved in hard work requires the aid of a doctor and other health-care professionals to make the journey toward recovery a safe one.

*   *   *

BE A CAVEMAN

Nothing is forcing you to recover. And that just may be the problem.

Archaeologists make their living describing how our distant ancestors lived. They have found many skeletons of early humans with bone fractures, amputations, and skull trauma. Archaeologists have also found evidence of arthritis, as well as an assortment of other injuries and illness. In many cases, these early humans survived their injuries. It can be assumed that these distant ancestors also had strokes. If a member of a tribal community had a stroke, their "therapy" would be ferocious. Survival of the tribe and the stroke survivor would dictate their "caveman therapy." Efforts toward recovery would focus on walking because these early humans were hunter-gatherers and they needed to move quickly in search of food. Stroke survivors would have had to learn to feed themselves or go hungry, toilet or get bacterial infections, and walk or get left behind. Sheer survival dictated the tremendous amount of energy they put into their recovery efforts. Their rehabilitation would flow organically from what they knew they had to do.

No doubt, their recovery from stroke would be physically demanding. But they would have been used to huge amounts of hard physical work. Every day of their prestroke lives was a struggle *for* food, and *against* the elements, beasts, and the threat of starvation. Walking long distances, hunting, hut building, tool making, rudimentary sewing, foraging, and so forth, would have made these humans tough beyond modern understanding. In that sense, stroke survivors today are at a disadvantage. We've gone soft. Are we able to channel the toughness that hides deep in our shared DNA?

Along with a physical toughness, these ancestors would have had another advantage: They were forced to recover. No other member of the tribe would be able to speak as loudly as his or her own inner voice. "I will survive." The end result of this raging recovery would be more recovery than similar stroke survivors experience today. Much of this concept is covered in research under the term, **task-specific training**. Research has found that:

- If you practice a movement, you might get better at that movement.
- If you practice that same movement as part of a real-world task, you can expect more recovery.
- If you practice the movement within a real-world environment that is important to you, you can expect even more return of movement.
- If you practice a task that is vital to you, you will get the most return of movement.

The more vital the task is, the more you will be driven toward recovery. Early humans would have viewed almost everything they did, every day of their lives, as vital. Their tasks were more than just important, they were *essential* to survival. Their bones whisper the secret of recovery: *Work on recovery as if your life depends on it.*

HOW IS IT DONE?

Some stroke survivors use something close to this "caveman therapy." People who obtain the best recovery from stroke tend to be people who *have* to get better. Their life goals dictate that they must recover. They challenge themselves in ways that other stroke survivors don't. Driving their recovery are passions like independence, career, or essential hobbies like playing piano, painting, or pool. These modern-day "cavemen" and "cavewomen" are rare. They reclaim their passions because *their life depends on it.*

The most effective clinical therapies mimic this recovery strategy. These therapies attempt to *force* recovery in one way or another. They are designed to cajole, prompt, and encourage but they are, in the end, artificial. Researchers have been obsessed with designing artificial motivation. They try virtual reality, video gaming, and an assortment of other gizmos and tricks. But there is no substitute for that feeling from which recovery flows. What is it that you love? What in your life *must* you do? What do you have left to accomplish? Focus on these activities to unleash your inner caveman.

WHAT PRECAUTIONS SHOULD BE TAKEN?

If skiing is your passion and you need to get back on your skis, don't just strap them on and head for the mountain. Include your doctor, therapists, family, and friends in your plans, and train safely as you move toward your goal. You are not a caveman. Your responsibility to your own recovery requires that you stay safe.

*   *   *

WHEN HELP HURTS

Life's day-to-day challenges present opportunities to work on recovery. Think about the devices you use to improve your life. Consider reducing any form of assistance that is not essential to safety and/or independence. Doing so will open up a world of productive struggle.

Assistive devices (ADs) and the broader term **adaptive equipment** are names for rehabilitation gear that:

- Makes your life easier
- Makes you safer
- Helps you be more independent in your daily life

Examples of these devices include:

- Specialized eating utensils
- Wheelchairs
- Reachers
- Leg lifters
- Zipper and button aids
- Writing aids
- Ambulatory aids (canes, walkers, etc.).
- Splints (ankle-foot orthosis, hand splints, etc.)

Assistive devices can promote independence, make your life easier, and make everyday living safer. But they may have a downside, too. These devices can make tasks that should be a challenge, easier. Doing without an AD can promote recovery. The challenge inherent in everyday tasks is important to the process of recovery from stroke. It is worthwhile to weigh all the advantages of the AD, with special consideration regarding safety issues.

The typical medical model assumes that recovery from stroke is best served by making you safe, comfortable, and making life as easy as possible. *"Treat 'em and street 'em"* is often the mantra and if "streeting 'em" requires a few helpful ADs, well then why not? There are actually good reasons for thinking this way. The stroke survivor, his or her family, and the insurance company decide the speed at which survivors are pushed through the system. Simply, the goal is to get you as independent as possible in the shortest amount of time possible. Part of this effort involves providing the necessary

AD to speed up the process. But there are points in the arc of recovery where you should question the need for individual ADs. Keep in mind that an AD can mask the fact that you can do without the device. With every AD you use, you are asked to do less and are discouraged from doing more. Attempting less generally means less recovery. An ongoing and thoughtful evaluation of the necessity of all ADs is wise.

Consider pens with a built-up barrel. These "fat pens" have been used by stroke survivors for the same reason small children use oversized pencils: The fatter a writing utensil, the easier it is to control. When you use an oversized pen, you require less of your fingers. This continual lack of challenge reduces the chance of ever gripping regular pens and pencils. Coordination and dexterity are challenged less. The fine-motor aspect of gripping is not challenged, so all the tasks that require the same sort of grasp will suffer. Larger utensils should be used temporarily as you progress toward more challenging grasping tasks. But many survivors use these aids for the rest of their lives.

If the AD does not impact safety, then eliminating it becomes a decision based on its relative necessity versus the therapeutic value of not using it.

Here are two other ADs that should be reconsidered:

- Hand splints neither improve movement nor reduce **contracture**. Splints give the false impression that the splint is doing all the work that is needed. Splinting eliminates the use of muscles that control the splinted joints. Immobilizing joints in this way will reduce the amount of brain dedicated to those joints. This causes a sort of "reverse **neuroplasticity**." This reduces the amount of brainpower to those same joints, muscles, and movements that you're trying to recover. Splints also discourage stretching of all the joints on the affected hand through their full **range of motion**. The "bad" hand is especially vulnerable when not stretched because of the many joints involved. Soft tissue can shorten on the palm side of the fingers, leaving fingers forever fisted. Some splints, especially off-the-shelf splints, can actually damage the joints in the hand by forcing the hand into unnatural positions. This can cause small tears in the joints of the hand and fingers.
- An **ankle-foot orthosis** (**AFO**) stabilizes the ankle and raises the foot during walking when the leg is swinging forward. The AFO

makes walking easier, but less is being required of the foot and leg. The foot is no longer being asked to lift (dorsiflex) at the ankle. Also, less is required in terms of coordination of the entire "bad" leg and foot. There are good reasons for using AFOs, including important safety issues. However, if your doctor agrees and if walking can be done safely, the extra effort may pay off in:

— Strengthening of the muscles that lift the foot
— Increased coordination during lifting the foot
— Strengthening of the muscles stabilizing the ankle
— A larger area of brain cells dedicated to the ankle (**neuroplasticity**)
— Increased ability to move the ankle
— More challenge toward normal coordination of the entire "bad" leg and foot

Note: Do not end the use of splinting or an AFO without the consent and sanction of your doctor. Ending use of an AFO can lead to falls.

HOW IS IT DONE?

There are two broad ways to gradate the use of an assistive device (AD):

1. Increasing or decreasing the *time* the device is used
2. Increasing or decreasing the *type* of device, so there is more or less assistance

Some examples of gradation of dosage include:

• Choosing to begin to use the AD
• Increasing the amount of time that you use the AD
• Reducing the amount of time that you use the AD
• Ending the use of the AD

Some examples of gradation of type include:

• Examples of gradation of the amount of support used for walking
— A walker (a lot of support)
— Hemi-cane
— Quad cane
— Straight cane (a little support)
— No walking aid (no support)

- Examples of gradation of aids used to lift the foot and stabilize the ankle
  — Ankle-foot orthosis
  — Ankle brace or ankle stabilizer
  — Flexible (e.g., Neoprene) ankle wrap
  — High-top athletic shoes
  — Shoes
  — Walking barefoot
- Decreasing the size of a "build up" (widening the circumference) on a writing or eating utensil
- Reducing the use or eliminating elastic shoelaces, buttoning, and zipping aids

This list represents just a few of a long and growing list of ADs used by stroke survivors. Occupational and physical therapists can provide a full list of available ADs.

WHAT PRECAUTIONS SHOULD BE TAKEN?

The safety implications of ending your relationship with ADs can be enormous.

If the AD does impact safety, then a much more vigorous and thoughtful consideration must be taken. Ending usage of some ADs has the potential of putting the stroke survivor in danger. Consult with your doctor regarding ending use of any AD or splint. *Do not end the use of splinting or an AFO without the consent and sanction of your doctor.*

Also, it may be that you are not using an AD that you should be using. An AD can promote safety, independence, and/or promote recovery. New ADs are being developed and put on the market every day. Assistive devices may provide efficiency and safety. They can also be an interim step on your road toward recovery. Some ADs have no downside, and that contain great benefits. For instance, grab-bars in the bathroom keep you safe in slippery areas where challenging balance is dangerous.

RECONSIDER MEDICATIONS

Rule One: DON'T EVER STOP TAKING MEDICATIONS OR CHANGE DOSAGES WITHOUT DISCUSSING IT WITH YOUR DOCTOR!

Rule Two: DON'T EVER STOP TAKING MEDICATIONS OR CHANGE DOSAGES WITHOUT DISCUSSING IT WITH YOUR DOCTOR!

Rule Three: SEE RULES ONE AND TWO.

Drugs affect your recovery. Drugs include all medications that are prescribed, over-the-counter, or in foods (e.g., caffeine). Drugs affect everyone physically, emotionally, and/or mentally. Stroke survivors have the extra burden of trying to figure out how their medications affect their recovery efforts.

Therapists have always viewed their client's medications as a mixed blessing. Consider oral antispasticity drugs. They reduce spasticity, which helps make movement easier. But these medications are designed to relax muscles. When taken orally, these drugs are nonspecific. That is, they do not just target muscles that are spastic, they relax *all* muscles. Because they affect all muscles, they tend to make patients tired. A tired patient cannot put her full mental and physical effort into her recovery. Pain pills, psychotropic medications (drugs that affect the mind), sleeping pills, and other drugs can have similar (tiring and/or unmotivating) results. Drugs can help or hurt your recovery effort. In fact, from one day to the next, the same medication may be a benefit and then a detriment. For example, narcotic pain medications. On Monday it may be too painful for you to move without the medication, so the drug is beneficial to recovery. On Tuesday you have little pain but the medication has made you so tired that you can't focus on doing the physical movement required in therapy.

Sometimes adding a new medication helps recovery. A stroke survivor, here called "Tim," had excruciating pain in his affected arm. Tim had what is called shoulder-hand syndrome. This is a form of reflex sympathetic dystrophy (RSD), a problem in up to 25% of stroke survivors. Tim asked his doctor what he could do to rehab his arm and hand. "Nothing," the doctor answered. "Not until the pain can be reduced." His doctor then suggested

that Tim see a physiatrist. The physiatrist correctly diagnosed his pain and
gave him a new medication that dramatically decreased the pain. This meant
Tim could finally move his arm in relative comfort, and efforts toward recovery could then begin.

The decision of which drugs should be used and should not be used is
best left between you and your doctor.

HOW IS IT DONE?

A frank discussion with your doctor about the impact of medications on
your recovery is prudent at any and all points during the arc of recovery.

WHAT PRECAUTIONS SHOULD BE TAKEN?

Again, *never* discontinue medications or change dosages without discussing it thoroughly with your doctor!

*   *   *

FIGHT FATIGUE

Severe fatigue affects up to 70% of stroke survivors. Many survivors
consider fatigue to be the worst symptom caused by the stroke. Fatigue im-
pedes recovery. Adopting strategies that help reduce fatigue is essential to
achieving recovery goals. There are many reasons for fatigue after stroke,
including:

- A lot of tiring therapy
- Everyday activities that can use 100% more energy than they did
  prior to the stroke
- Stress from life after stroke that saps energy and makes sleeping
  more difficult
- Prescribed medications that often add to fatigue
- Muscular weakness
- Cardiovascular weakness

In some stroke survivors, the following may also cause, or add to, fatigue:

- Pain
- Depression
- Living alone
- Living in an institution
- Having trouble speaking or understanding

Post-stroke fatigue creates a downward spiral of disability. The more fatigue, the less effort is made toward cardiovascular and muscle strengthening. Decreased levels of exercise lead to weight gain, which leads to greater effort needed to move. This, in turn, leads to more fatigue, which leads to less exercise...and the spiral continues. It is a classic Catch-22: if you want more energy, you have to exercise, but in order to exercise you need energy.

Fatigue impacts many aspects of a stroke survivor's life, not the least of which is his recovery. It goes without saying that, if you are too tired to fully engage in your recovery effort, less progress will be made.

HOW IS IT DONE?

Here are some suggestions to help reduce fatigue, so that maximal effort can be devoted to recovery:

- *As unbelievable as it may seem, exercise actually reduces fatigue,* even in the short term. Yes, exercise fights fatigue!
- *Increase your muscular strength.* The more stored strength your muscles have, the less the fatigue you will experience.
- *Increase your cardiovascular strength.* The more stored energy your heart and lungs have, the less fatigue you will experience.
- *Meditate.* Stress saps needed energy. Meditation can reduce stress.
- *Reconsider your medications.* Some medications reduce energy. These medications can include psychotropic (drugs that affect the mind) and spasticity medications. On the other hand, other medications are stimulants. These drugs increase energy, at least in the short term. (Warning: do not ever stop taking medications or change dosages without discussing it with your doctor!)
- *Stroke causes brain damage.* Brain damage caused by stroke can disrupt normal sleep cycles. Some survivors have found that periods of

rest and/or regular naps can help. Some research has shown that naps actually lower the risk of dying of heart disease and stroke. However, unintentionally falling asleep, or dozing, is actually an indicator for future strokes. People who fall asleep unintentionally have a four to five times greater risk of stroke than folks who don't doze. On the other hand, dozing is an effect of being tired. So sleeping well at night is the best answer. "Early to bed and early to rise, makes a man healthy, wealthy, and wise" is a quote by Benjamin Franklin. He may as well have been talking about the positive effect of adequate sleep on stroke recovery. The sleeping habits of humans were developed over hundreds of thousands of years of evolution. People are "programmed" to go to bed when the sun goes down and wake up as the sun rises. Artificial lighting, TV, and computers are just a few devices that trick your brain into thinking it is daytime, even during the night. Sleeping habits that involve going to bed at a set hour help add consistency and often allow for adequate rest.

- *Proper nutrition can increase energy.* Eating refined carbohydrates (white breads, pastries, rice, pasta, donuts, bagels candy, soda, etc.) can reduce energy. Fresh fruits and vegetables and lean protein choices can increase energy.
- *Drink plenty of water.* Dehydration saps energy. As people age, the sense of thirst decreases, so drink water even when you aren't "dying of thirst."

Some people believe that the best way to reduce fatigue after stroke is to make life as easy as possible. But overcoming the physical challenges presented after stroke has great therapeutic value. Ironically, *overcoming the challenges left in the wake of a stroke is the best way to recover from stroke.* However, sometimes energy-saving devices and strategies are necessary and actually help the process of recovery. A balance needs to be maintained between making life too easy, and making life so hard that you don't have the energy to recover.

WHAT PRECAUTIONS SHOULD BE TAKEN?

All of the suggestions for fighting fatigue should be done under the supervision of your doctor. There are many medical reasons for fatigue, from dehydration to diabetes, and from pain to depression. It is essential that the underlying cause of fatigue be determined.

✻ ✻ ✻

WALKING YOUR WAY TO BETTER WALKING

As obvious as it sounds, the best way of improving the quality of walking is to walk. The act of walking uses some of the most progressive concepts in recent rehabilitation research. For instance, one of the techniques researchers use to promote robust recovery is called **task-specific training**. This means training for recovery within the context of a valued task. There are few tasks more valued than walking. Walking also involves another buzz concept in rehab research: **repetitive practice** (the same movement is repeated). Researchers believe repetitive practice is essential to relearning a skill. Another cutting-edge concept in stroke rehabilitation is adding a **rhythmic** component. Walking is inherently rhythmic. Walking also involves another rehabilitation concept that researchers are keen on: **bilateral training**. Bilateral training involves having the two legs communicating with each other. Researchers believe that the two arms and two legs communicate with each other in two ways:

- The limbs communicate through the brain.
- The limbs communicate directly, right through the spinal cord, without the brain involved.

So walking brings together four advanced concepts:

1. Task specificity: This involves practicing exactly what is to be learned.
2. Repetitive: This involves doing the same movement over and over.
3. **Rhythmicity**: This involves adding a beat. Walking itself supplies the beat.
4. Bilateral training: This is where the two legs communicate directly. During bilateral training, the "good" limb can make the "bad" limb move better and faster.

Walking may just be the best exercise available. Walking:

- Is "low impact," so it puts little stress on the joints
- "Banks" energy for the heart and lungs
- Burns calories and controls weight
- Controls blood sugar
- Increases mental agility
- Decreases the chance of blood clots in the legs, which reduces the risk of another stroke
- Builds muscle
- Improves balance and may decrease falls
- Increases bone strength

... and much more.

HOW IS IT DONE?

There are a lot of ways to stay safe while pursuing an aggressive walking program. Proper orthotics, such as an **ankle-foot orthosis (AFO)** and appropriate walking aids, such as canes and walkers, can be discussed with your doctor and physical therapist. If, however, you are not yet ready to walk without support, there are still options (beyond wearing a gait belt and having therapists help you). All of the following are done under the care of a physical therapist:

- **Treadmill training** (TT). This can provide the safety and comfort of walking indoors with the added safety benefit of providing "endless parallel bars." Treadmill training has inherent risks that can lead to falling. See page 25 for full details on treadmill training.
- **Partial weight supported walking (PWSW)** .
  - *PWSW on a treadmill*: You are partially supported by a harness. The harness can be raised to reduce the amount of weight you're carrying. The harness can also be lowered so that you are carrying your full weight, but the harness catches you if you fall. This allows you to challenge your balance without risk of falls. The product usually associated with this type of training is called the LiteGait®.
  - *PWSW over ground*: This system is the same as the treadmill version except you walk over flat ground. Products that fall into this category include the Biodex Unweighing System, the NeuroGym® Bungee Walker, and the LiteGait®. Contact a physical

therapist or local rehabilitation hospital to find facilities in your area that provide PWSW.

- Researchers have found great results with a new kind of gait (walking) therapy. It is called speed-intensive gait training (SIGT). Speed-intensive gait training is a simple idea; your walking will get better and faster if you practice walking faster. Walking faster improves the quick movements needed to control balance, which translates into smoother and more efficient walking. And SIGT has been used to double the walking speed of study participants. Speed-intensive gait training may or may not involve weight support as in PWSW.

WHAT PRECAUTIONS SHOULD BE TAKEN?

Walking is one of the most natural movements humans perform. But a walking regimen designed to improve the quality of gait takes more physical and mental effort than leisure walking. Because this type of walking regime is more intense than leisure walking, make sure to talk to your doctor and therapist prior to incorporating therapeutic walking into a total rehabilitation plan. If you are able to walk without aid, do so with safety in mind. Your doctor and therapist will provide the medical and physical limits that should be observed.

Recovery Machines

THOSE AMAZING MACHINES

Many researchers, medical doctors, and bioengineers dedicate much of their career and cash to the development and marketing of stroke-recovery machines. Why do they spend so much time and money on stroke recovery? Because there are 50 million stroke survivors worldwide, and it's a global economy. If an inventor brings one product to market and sells that product to just a small fraction of the 50 million, he stands to make a fortune. The tremendous potential for profit drives recovery machine development. This is promising news for stroke survivors. Many machines are already on the market, and more are on their way. It is wise for survivors to consider recovery machines now available, and keep an eye on emerging stroke-recovery technologies.

Deciding which machines are appropriate for your recovery can be tricky. Much like picking and choosing other recovery options, picking machines is a matter of deciding what fits with:

- Where you are in recovery
- What you need to accomplish
- How much you can afford

Stroke-recovery technology can be expensive. On the other hand, some of these machines are designed to go home with you. This provides the opportunity for you to expand and magnify your at-home recovery effort without the ongoing aid of clinicians. In the long run, this can save time and money.

Many machines can help jump start a new phase in recovery. Other machines lessen the humdrum of **repetitive practice** by turning repetitive movements into a game. Some machines build muscle, some teach spastic muscles to relax, some encourage improved coordination, some help develop cardiovascular strength, and so forth. From walking to swallowing, and from visual deficits to speech impairments, there are machines that attempt to treat every movement deficit caused by stroke.

HOW IS IT DONE?

The following list provides broad categories of stroke-recovery technologies. Included are general explanations of what machines in those categories do.

- *Cyclic electrical stimulation.* Cyclic electrical stimulation (**e-stim**) machines send electrical stimulation through electrodes to the skin overlying the muscles you want to work. This sort of e-stim may jump start movement in paralyzed muscles. It may also build bulk and strength in paralyzed muscles. Also, e-stim may relax muscles that are spastic by stimulating the muscles antagonistic (opposite) to the spastic muscles.
- *Electromyography (EMG)-based electrical stimulation (e-stim) with biofeedback.* These are e-stim machines with another feature added: The machine senses the effort of your muscles. If you tighten the muscle enough, you reach a threshold. Once you reach the threshold, the machine helps you complete the movement you are attempting. This process, called **biofeedback**, turns the passive activity provided by cyclic e-stim into an active exercise. Brain rewiring (**neuroplasticity**) is believed to occur because mental and/or physical effort is required.
- *E-stim orthotics.* These orthotics are worn on the recovering limbs. They differ from other forms of e-stim because they do not just "turn on and turn off" muscles. Instead, these orthotics stimulate muscles in the right way to do some real-world task. For instance, some e-stim orthotics lift the foot for people with **foot drop**. There are arm/hand orthotics that will help you open and close your hand, so you can grasp and release objects. These orthotics have the advantage of working on two levels:

  - They help you do some real-world task (e.g., grasping an object, walking, etc.). This **task-specific** training can promote recovery in that limb.
  - They encourage you to use the joints around the orthotic. For instance, an orthotic worn on the forearm and hand will also promote movement in the shoulder and elbow. In the leg, an orthotic that helps lift the foot will encourage improved movement from the hip and knee.

  Unlike other forms of electrical stimulation, e-stim orthotics have the electrodes built in, eliminating or reducing the number of wires that tether the user to the machine.
- *Electromyography-based gaming.* These types of games work by sending information from muscles into a machine. These signals travel to the machine and guide a character or other game element on the

screen. The machine uses your muscular effort to play a variety of video games from solitaire to pinball.

- *Virtual reality (VR) gaming* (see You Are Game—Virtual Reality, page 87). The biggest news in VR gaming for stroke survivors is the release of the Wii system by Nintendo. This system allows you to move images on a TV screen by moving a hand-held controller. Virtual reality gaming provides a safe, challenging, and fun environment in which to recover. Beyond the Wii system, many VR systems are inexpensive and plug directly into any TV with RCA-type inputs. Therapists have even named this therapy: Wii-habilitation!

- *Bilateral arm trainers*. **Bilateral training** (BT) does not require equipment of any kind. For instance, walking is a form of BT. With every stride, the "good" leg provides guidance to the "bad" side about proper position and timing. There are machines that promote BT, however. Upper-extremity ergometers (stationary cycles used with arms or legs) are examples of simple bilateral trainers. Others include hand-crank upper-body ergometers, stationary bicycles, recumbent bilateral exercisers with arm components, and so forth.

- *Body weight-supported treadmill trainers*. A treadmill has many assets as a tool for relearning how to walk (see page 26). One of the ways to safely use a treadmill, even for folks still unable to walk, is to support the weight of the body with a harness. These systems reduce the effect of gravity and also keep you safe if there is a loss of balance. Called partial weight-supported treadmill training (PWSW), this relatively low-tech safety apparatus is available at many rehabilitation hospitals. Some stroke survivors don't yet have the coordination to bring the "bad" leg forward while involved in PWSW. The assistance, if needed to move the leg forward, can be provided by therapists crouched at the side of the treadmill. They literally grab the foot and leg and lift it off the ground to push it into the next step. The newer version of this technology has replaced therapists' hard work with a machine that moves the leg. An example of this sort of machine is the Lokomat®. Leg cuffs are attached to the hips, legs, ankles, and feet. The computer-driven leg cuffs progress the legs and feet in a way that promotes normal gait. This technology is quite expensive but is sometimes available at rehabilitation hospitals and other rehabilitation facilities. PWSW, when therapists assist leg movement, is much more low-tech. All that's needed is a treadmill and a harness. It can, however, be labor intensive if a therapist is needed to progress the foot during stepping.

- *Body weight-supported trainers without treadmills.* These trainers are weight support systems that allow you to carry less of your own weight as you relearn walking. A rolling platform suspends you while you walk on the floor. The amount of weight supported can be increased or decreased so, as you develop greater balance, the machine takes less of your weight. These machines include the NeuroGym® Bungee Walker, the Biodex Unweighing System, and the KineAssist™.
- *Cardiovascular machines.* Cardiovascular strength (stamina) directly impacts the amount and speed of recovery. Machines that increase stamina include treadmills, the NuStep®, and BioStep® **bilateral** trainer. Cardiovascular exercise is vital to recovery from stroke.

With any technology you use consider the following:

- Ease of use
- Cost
- If it needs a therapist or doctor to implement
- If it can be used at home
- If there is a substantial amount of clinical research that shows positive results

Stroke-Recovery Machines and What They Do

A list of stroke-recovery machines with descriptions and contact information follows. *The descriptions of these machines (in italics) were taken directly from the manufacturer and do not represent an endorsement by the author or the publisher.*

Contact information can always be found on the website. The website will be the quickest, easiest, and maybe even the best source of information on these machines. If you, your doctor, or your treating therapist have any questions about acquiring and/or using the machine, the manufacturer is the best resource. Generally speaking, the manufacturer will know the most about:

- Cost
- If are available lease options
- Insurance coverage (if any)

- Where to find the machine
- What research has been done on the machine
- If the machine is appropriate for your deficits
- Which therapists in your area are trained to use the machine

This section has three parts:

1. Machine names and website(s) (if available) are listed.
2. In italics, find what the machine does, in the words of the manufacturer.
3. The STATUS section tells if the machines are commercially available and if the stroke survivor can use them without help, or with supervision from a clinician.

Machines that help arm and hand movement and function

- H200™ (www.bionessinc.com) *The H200 is a non-invasive device, worn on the forearm and hand that enables patients to perform every day activities that were previously impossible. The NESS H200 can help the hand open and close, reduce stiffness, increase range of motion and strength, improve circulation and assist in regaining awareness of an impaired limb. In addition to the amazing therapeutic benefits of the H200, patients have also embraced the comfort and ease of use of the system. Unlike other systems, the H200 orthosis incorporates a self-adjusting fit, to hold the wrist and hand in a functional position. This superior fit, coupled with the H200 electrode placement, allows patients to remove and replace the device without compromising therapy effectiveness. Also, the patented technology behind the H200 provides six different stimulation patterns to enable patients to perform a variety of tasks and use it for therapeutic activities as well. The system is also versatile enough to be used in varied settings-including the home, with little technical expertise needed.*
  — STATUS: Commercially available. A therapist or physician should always supervise this treatment at the beginning. However, with training, this treatment can be done at home by the stroke survivor.

- Myomo™ (www.myomo.com) *Myomo therapy does not require invasive procedures or electrical stimulation of any kind. Rather, Myomo incorporates its noninvasive neurorobotic platform technology in wear-*

able, portable lightweight devices that are designed to enable patient-initiated-and-controlled motion. The wearable, portable, lightweight robotic brace slides onto the arm. By sensing the patient's electrical muscle activity through electromyography (EMG)-which detects muscle cells' electrical activity when they contract-and sending that data to a motor, it allows stroke patients to control their affected limbs. When used under the supervision of an occupational or physical therapist, the device can be used to help patients progress from basic motor training, such as lifting boxes or reaching for a light switch, to more complex tasks such as carrying a laundry basket or flipping a light on and off while holding an object with the unaffected limb.

— STATUS: The Myomo e100 is cleared only for clinical use at this time, meaning that it must be implemented by a therapist or physician.

- Armeo® (www.hocoma.com) *The Armeo facilitates intensive task-oriented upper extremity therapy after stroke, traumatic brain injury or other neurological diseases and injuries. It combines an adjustable arm support, with augmented feedback and a large 3-D workspace that allows functional therapy exercises in a virtual reality environment.*

— STATUS: Not yet available in the United States.

- Hand Mentor™ (www.handmentor.com or www.columbiasci. com) *The Hand Mentor™ is the first Active Repetitive Motion™ hand therapy device designed for use in therapy clinics to improve outcomes in stroke rehabilitation. The Hand Mentor™ actively involves the patient in their rehabilitation by encouraging self-initiated motion in the wrist and fingers, and assisting movement only when necessary.*

— STATUS: The "Pro" version, for treatment by therapists, will is clinically available. The manufacturer is in the process of engineering an at-home version of the Hand Mentor™.

- SaeboFlex® (www.SaeboFlex.com) *The SaeboFlex positions the wrist and fingers into extension in preparation for functional activities. The user is able to grasp an object by voluntarily flexing his or her fingers. The extension spring system assists in re-opening the hand to release the object. Saebo equipment, especially the SaeboFlex orthosis, is specialized patented technology. Occupational and physical therapists attend specific education classes offered by Saebo, Inc. to become trained in the SaeboFlex.*

— STATUS: Commercially available. A therapist or physician always supervises this treatment in the beginning. However, with training, there is potential for this treatment to be done by the stroke survivor, at home.

- Reo™ Go (www.motorika.com) *The Reo Go is a portable, easy to use system for delivering Reo Therapy. Combining streamlined ergonomic design and advanced software, the Reo Go provides a robust platform for highly effective robot-assisted upper extremity therapy.*
  — STATUS: Commercially available. A therapist or physician should always supervise this treatment. This machine is expensive. However, treatment on this machine may not cost any more than typical physical-therapy treatments.

- STIMuGRIP® (www.finetech-medical.co.uk/product-hand.htm) *The STIMuGRIP® system is designed to restore control of the wrist extension and hand grasp functions to users following a stroke or neurological insult. The system consists of an external controller, which is worn on the forearm over the site of the implanted internal parts. The controller contains sensors for triggering the pre-programmed stimulation routines and provides a simple interface for the user to select the appropriate routine.*
  — STATUS: Commercially available.

Machines that help leg and foot and walking

- NESS L300™ (www.bionessinc.com) *The NESS L300 utilizes proprietary technology that not only lets you walk smoother, but faster as well. And, only the NESS L300 has a built in sensor that recognizes the surface you are walking on and adjusts accordingly. It is also a much more streamlined device compared to other available options. There are no bulky wires to deal with and the compact design even allows patients to wear their normal footwear. It's also easy for patients to use. Unlike some systems, that can't easily be taken off and on, the NESS L300 is surprisingly simple-making it ideal for inpatient or outpatient use.*
  — STATUS: Commercially available. A medical doctor or physical therapist supervises this treatment. However, the stroke survivor can also use this treatment at home during everyday walking.

- WalkAide (www.walkaide.com) *WalkAide uses advanced sensor technology to actually analyze the movement of your leg and foot. The system*

sends electrical signals to your peroneal nerve, which controls movement in your ankle and foot. These gentle electrical impulses activate the muscles to raise your foot at the appropriate time during the step cycle.
— STATUS: Commercially available. This treatment is supervised by a medical doctor or physical therapist. However, the stroke survivor can also use this treatment at home during everyday walking.

- Odstock Dropped Foot Stimulator (ODFS) (www.odstockmedical.com) *The Odstock Dropped Foot Stimulator (ODFS) …is a pocket size medical device that helps to lift the dropped foot whilst walking. It applies small pulses of electrical stimulation to the nerves of the affected muscle, causing the muscle to contract and the foot to lift. The stimulation is applied to the outside of the leg using self adhesive patches called electrodes. The muscle contraction is timed to walking using a small switch placed inside the shoe. This technique is known as Functional Electrical Stimulation (FES).*
    — STATUS: Commercially available. This treatment is supervised by a medical doctor or physical therapist. However, the stroke survivor can also use this treatment at home during everyday walking.

- STIMuSTEP™ (www.odstockmedical.com) *The STIMuSTEP is an implanted neuromuscular stimulator intended for the correction of dropped foot following an upper motor-neurone lesion. While providing the same function as the ODFS, the device removes the need to accurately place electrodes each day, reduces the sensation of the stimulation and improves the convenience for the user. The device can only be supplied after initial successful trials or usage of an external ODFS unit.*
    — STATUS: Commercially available. A medical doctor always performs this treatment. However, the stroke survivor may use this treatment at home during everyday walking, while a medical doctor and therapist continue to monitor the treatment.

- LiteGait® (www.litegait.com) *LiteGait® is a therapy device used to promote the generation of normal walking patterns by controlling weight bearing, balance and posture during walking therapy.*
    — STATUS: Commercially available. A therapist or physician always supervises this treatment.

- NeuroGym® Bungee Walker (www.neurogymtech.com) *The Neuro-Gym® Bungee Walker is a versatile body weight support mechanism enabling safe, intensive motor retraining. The unique patented design enables the re-training of gait and natural protective reactions by counteracting loss of stability as naturally as possible. Comparable to a pool environment in terms of support, the Bungee Walker allows graduated weight bearing while normal protective reactions such as sidestepping are re-developed.*
  — STATUS: Commercially available. A therapist or physician always supervises this treatment in the beginning. However, with training, there is potential for this treatment to be done by the stroke survivor at home.

- Biodex Unweighing System (www.biodex.com/rehab) *The Biodex Unweighing System enables partial weight-bearing therapy to be conducted with the assurance of patient comfort and safety, and with convenient access to the patient for manual assistance and observation.*
  — STATUS: Commercially available. A therapist or physician always supervises this treatment in the beginning. However, with training, there is potential for this treatment to be done by the stroke survivor at home.

- Gait Trainer 2™ (www.biodex.com/rehab) *The Gait Trainer 2™ is the only treadmill with an instrumented deck that monitors and records step length, step speed and right-to-left time distribution (step symmetry). Patients are motivated by the real-time audio and visual biofeedback. They are prompted into proper gait patterns; step length, step speed and step symmetry.*
  — STATUS: Commercially available. A therapist or physician always supervises this treatment in the beginning. However, with training, there is potential for this treatment to be done by the stroke survivor at home.

- Lokomat® (www.hocoma.com) *Locomotion therapy supported by an automated gait orthosis on a treadmill has established itself as an effective intervention for improving over-ground walking function caused by neurological diseases and injuries. The Lokomat is the first driven gait orthosis that assists walking movements of gait-impaired patients and is used to improve mobility in individuals following stroke, spinal cord injury, traumatic brain injury, multiple sclerosis or other neurological diseases and injuries.*

— STATUS: Commercially available. A therapist or physician always supervises this treatment. This machine is very expensive. However, treatment on this machine may not cost any more than typical physical therapy treatments.

- Reo Ambulator (www.motorika.com) *Reo Ambulator is an innovative robotic gait training device that integrates body weight support treadmill training (BWSTT) with advanced robotics to help rehabilitate patients who experience neuromuscular dysfunction to address problems with ambulation, balance, coordination, posture and stamina.*
  — STATUS: Commercially available. A therapist or physician always supervises this treatment. This machine is very expensive. However, treatment on this machine may not cost any more than typical physical therapy treatments.

- KineAssist™ (www.kineadesign.com/portfolio/kineassist) *KineAssist™ technology will allow therapists to safely challenge patients in functional environments with reduced concern about falls, record objective measures and integrate with existing practice settings.*
  — STATUS: Commercially available. A therapist or physician always supervises this treatment.

Machines that can be used for the upper or lower extremities

- Neuromove™ (www.neuromove.com) *The NeuroMove™ works by detecting the attempts to move a muscle group sent from the brain. These attempts are shown in the display as significant increases in the signal over regular muscle activity. The built-in microprocessor intelligently distinguishes between regular muscle activity, muscle tone, noise and real attempts. When a real attempt is detected, the unit "rewards" the patient with a few seconds of muscle contraction, where the visual and sensory feedback serves as an important element in relearning the movement.*
  — STATUS: Commercially available. A therapist or physician always supervises this treatment in the beginning. However, with training, there is potential for this treatment to be done by the stroke survivor at home.

- Mentamove® (email: ryan@mentamove-na.com) *Electrodes are applied to the surface of your skin above the targeted muscle group. The electrodes measure the EMG, which is increased when you mentally practice a functional movement. The Mentamove® device then applies a comfortable electrical stimulation to activate the targeted muscle. This stimulation is activated mental activity alone.*

— STATUS: Commercially available. A therapist or physician always supervises this treatment in the beginning. However, with training, there is potential for this treatment to be done by the stroke survivor at home.

• The Biomove 3000 system (www.mystroke.com) *The system is able to detect the extremely small electrical EMG signals still measurable in paralyzed muscles after a stroke. These tiny signals are used to initiate an electrical stimulation impulse to the same muscles, resulting in actual muscle movement!*

— STATUS: Commercially available. A therapist or physician always supervises this treatment in the beginning. However, with training, there is potential for this treatment to be done by the stroke survivor at home.

• Core:Tx® (www.performancehealth.com) *The Core:Tx at home therapy program includes: easy-to-use software that guides you through therapy exercises; A wireless sensor that detects your movement when you wear it on your arm, leg, hand or foot with included gear; A base station that plugs into your home computer picks up the signal from the wireless sensor; A user guide with examples of exercises you can use to create your own therapy program at home.*

— STATUS: Commercially available. A therapist or physician always supervises this treatment in the beginning. However, with training, there is potential for this treatment to be done by the stroke survivor at home.

• Interactive Metronome (IM) (www.interactivemetronome.com) *The Interactive Metronome is an advanced brain-based treatment program designed to promote and enhance brain performance and recovery. This is accomplished by using innovative neurosensory and neuromotor exercises developed to improve the brain's inherent ability to repair or remodel itself through a process called neuroplasticity.*

— STATUS: Commercially available. A therapist or physician always supervises this treatment in the beginning. However, with training, there is potential for this treatment to be done by the stroke survivor at home.

Machines for other aspects of stroke recovery

- VitalStim Therapy (www.vitalstimtherapy.com) *VitalStim Therapy uses small electrical currents to stimulate the muscles responsible for swallowing. At the same time, trained specialists help patients "re-educate" their muscles through rehabilitation therapy.*
  — STATUS: Commercially available. A therapist or physician always supervises this treatment.

- NovaVision VRT™ Vision Restoration Therapy™ (www.novavision.com) *VRT is a clinically proven, FDA-cleared technology designed to improve the quality of life of stroke and brain injury patients by restoring some of their lost vision. The therapy does not require surgery or medication of any kind.*
  — STATUS: Commercially available. A therapist or physician always supervises this treatment. This machine is expensive. However, treatment on this machine may not cost any more than typical physical therapy treatments.

This list of machines is not complete, nor can it be. The rapid development of these new technologies means that new products become available every day.

FUTURE MACHINES

The best way to stay abreast of the latest and greatest recovery machines is to "keep your ear to the ground." Check the Internet, TV, and print for new ideas. The best outlet for information on cutting-edge machines for stroke rehabilitation is a website called Medgadget (www.medgadget.com/archives/rehab). The free magazines, *Stroke Smart* (www.strokesmart.org/) and *Stroke Connection* (www.strokeassociation.org), have great suggestions for new machines. The advertisements in these magazines provide a wealth of information, photographs, and contact information on commercially available stroke-recovery machines. There are also articles that review the latest stroke-recovery technology.

As time goes on, stroke recovery will rely more and more on machines. The most difficult part of this new machine-driven world of recovery is figuring out how to use these machines. Using some machines is as simple as placing a couple of electrodes and flipping a switch. Other machines are so complex that the machine is virtually useless. Some rehabilitation hospitals spend tens of thousands of dollars on machines that end up collecting dust. If the machine takes too long to learn, therapists won't use it. Also, if setting up the machine for a patient to use takes too long, then the machine will not be used. My hope, as we move forward, is that the folks who make these machines understand that simplicity of use is essential. If a machine is simple and effective, survivors will be inclined to buy it and use it at home. Or, if a therapist is needed, the machine needs to be simple enough to not burn available treatment time with a protracted set up.

WHAT PRECAUTIONS SHOULD BE TAKEN?

Make sure your doctor knows if you decide to add a machine to your recovery efforts. Some machines require a doctor's prescription. Contact individual manufacturers to determine if the machine needs a doctor's prescription. These machines may or may not be covered by insurance, depending on a number of factors. Again, the manufacturers will know if their machine is covered. They are in business to serve you, so you will find them helpful and informative as you consider their machine.

Recovery options that involve electrical stimulation have precautions and contraindications. Discuss these with your medical doctor prior to using any electrical stimulation options. Here is a partial list of contraindications and precautions for recovery options that use electrical stimulation:

- Pregnancy
- Skin irritation
- Epilepsy/ seizures
- Sensitive skin
- Compromised sensation
- Heart disease
- Pacemakers or defibrillators
- Recent surgery if muscle contraction may disrupt healing
- Electrode placement over the carotid sinus in the neck
- Existing thrombosis

Resources

The Evidence-Based Review of Stroke Rehabilitation (EBRSR) (website)

Website address: www.ebrsr.com.

The EBRSR is an easy way of accessing the latest and greatest that stroke-rehabilitation research has to offer. Each section (called a module) opens with an easily readable list that explains which therapies work, which ones do not work, and which are promising but still unproven. Not only that, but it is updated every 6 months.
Cost: Free

The StrokEngine (website)

Website address: www.medicine.mcgill.ca/Strokengine.

From acupuncture to virtual reality, the StrokEngine is called "the stroke rehabilitation intervention website." StrokEngine allows you to look up individual therapies to see if they hold promise for you. Once you've chosen a therapy, you can go to a section called Patient/Family Info. Once there, you can go to a section called Does It Work for Stroke? This section gets to the bottom line about that particular therapy.
Cost: Free

MedGadget (website)

Website address: http://medgadget.com/archives/rehab/

This website reviews the latest technology (machines) for stroke recovery.
Cost: Free

Google alerts

Website address: www.google.com/alerts

Google will email you any news stories about stroke recovery, depending on the search words you choose (i.e., "stroke recovery" and/or "stroke therapy," etc.). This is an easy way to stay abreast of advances in stroke-recovery techniques and technologies.
Cost: Free

The following two periodicals, both free, are invaluable to providing stroke survivors a window into new stroke-recovery options. You can subscribe by contacting them through their website or by phone.

Stroke Connection (magazine) (produced by the American Stroke Association)

Subscription Information:
Call: 1-888-478-7653.
Email: strokeconnection@heart.org
Website address: www.strokeassociation.org
Cost: Free

Stroke Smart (produced by the National Stroke Association)

Subscription Information
Call: 1-800-787-6537.
Website address: www.strokesmart.org
Cost: Free

If you are interested in getting therapy beyond what your insurance will provide, consider involvement in stroke-recovery research. Research trials often offer treatment options that are not available in any other clinical setting. There are research trials happening all over the country. Here are three Internet sites that have lists of ongoing trials.

Run by the National Institute of Health:

www.clinicaltrials.gov

Run by the Internet Stroke Center at Washington University School of Medicine:

www.strokecenter.org/trials

Run by CenterWatch, a business of Jobson Medical Information:

www.centerwatch.com

Google, the giant Internet search engine, also lists clinical trials. To access their list go to Google (www.google.com). In the search panel type in "clinical trials" and click the "Search" button. At the top of the next page it will say "Find results for clinical trials in Clinical trials search." Under this statement a pull down window in which you can type "stroke."

Glossary

Active movement

Movement done with the stroke survivor's own muscle power.

Active range of motion (AROM)

The arc of movement of a joint that the stroke survivor can perform with his own power.

Acute

The period immediately after stroke and continuing for 6 months to a year afterward. After the acute phase is the chronic phase. The chronic phase is usually considered to be the period from 6 months (or a year) after stroke until death.

Adaptive equipment

Any equipment that makes the life of stroke survivors easier or gives them the ability to do a task that they would not otherwise be able to do. This term tends to be used interchangeably with **assistive devices.**

AFO

See ankle-foot orthoses.

Ankle-foot orthoses (AFO)

An orthotic designed to lift the foot and stabilize the ankle during walking.

Aphasia

Aphasia is a general term for an inability or difficulty to either speak (expressive aphasia) or understand speech (receptive aphasia). Stroke survivors sometimes have aphasia when they have had a left-sided stroke (right side of the body affected).

Apraxic (apraxia)

An inability to plan movements. In stroke survivors, apraxia makes a movement difficult or impossible, even though they have the active range of motion (AROM) and strength to do it.

Assistive devices

Any equipment that makes the life of stroke survivors easier or gives them the ability to do a task that they would not otherwise be able to do. This term tends to be used interchangeably with the term **adaptive equipment.**

Balance training

Any recovery technique used to increase balance after stroke. Traditionally, balance training is done in a rehabilitation facility by a physical therapist.

Bilateral

Using either both of the upper or both of the lower extremities at the same time.

Bilateral training

Any recovery technique that involves repetitive and predictable patterned movement of either both of the upper extremities, or both of the lower extremities at the same time. Bilateral training falls into two main categories: 1) Equal and at the same time (as in conducting an orchestra) and (2) equal and alternating (as in drumming using alternating hands).

Biofeedback

A system that allows for a continuous monitoring of a body system in order to control that body system. Biofeedback happens all over the body all the time. For instance, in a simple biofeedback loop, to relax a muscle, you send signals to the muscle to contract and the muscle sends back a signal that tells you that the muscle is relaxed. Biofeedback is traditionally used to allow for control over systems in the body that are not normally controllable, like heart rate and blood pressure. In stroke survivors who want to move better, biofeedback can be used to monitor the contraction of a muscle or group of muscles that are not responding in order to encourage muscle contraction. An example of biofeedback used in stroke recovery is electromyography-based biofeedback machines.

Brunnstrom, Signe

Signe Brunnstrom, a Swedish Fulbright scholar and pioneer physical therapist was the first to map out the predictable **stages of recovery** from stroke. Although Hippocrates described stroke some 2,400 years earlier, Brunnstrom was the first to describe the landmarks on the road to recovery. These predictable stages of recovery are commonly called "Brunnstrom's stages of recovery." Some of the tests that Brunnstrom developed decades ago are still used in rehabilitation research, and the results of those tests tend to correlate well with more sophisticated computer-driven tests like testing of neuroplasticity by magnetic resonance imaging (MRI).

Brunnstrom's stages of recovery
The six predictable stages that stroke survivors experience during recovery from stroke. These stages go from Stage 1, in which the stroke survivor is flaccid to Stage 6, in which the stroke survivor is fully recovered.

Cardiovascular
Having to do with the heart and blood vessels. The term cardiovascular tends to be used to describe endurance of the heart and lungs.

Cardiovascular training
Training focused on increasing endurance of the heart and lungs.

Central obesity
Described as apple-shaped, this is a body shape where the waist is larger than the hips. This shape, as opposed to carrying weight around the hips, has been shown to have increased risk of high blood pressure, diabetes, heart disease, and stroke.

Chronic
The term used to describe a stroke survivor's time since stroke. The chronic stage after stroke is usually considered to be the period that is more than 6 months to a year after stroke. Before the chronic phase is the **acute** phase. The acute phase is usually considered to be the period immediately after stroke and continuing for 6 months to a year after stroke.

Compensatory movement
Relying on the unaffected limbs to do the activities of daily living.

Constraint-induced therapy (CIT) for the arm
Traditional CIT is a stroke-recovery technique that involves constraining the "good" arm and hand and having the stroke survivor only use the affected arm and hand in a clinical setting.

Constraint-induced therapy for the leg (leg CIT)
Four different schools of thought debate the exact definition of leg CIT: providing extensive and intensive exercises of the affected leg; partial weight-supported walking; electrical stimulation ankle-foot orthoses;

or providing a shoe lift or some other type of orthotic on the unaffected side, forcing weight onto the affected side.

Contracture

A shortening of soft tissue (e.g., muscle, nerves, blood vessels, etc.). A contracture happens when a joint is left flexed for too long and the soft tissue shortens. In stroke survivors, contracture happens in response to spastic muscles, which are in a constant state of contraction.

Conventional therapy

The usual care offered in a particular setting. After stroke, survivors are usually offered conventional therapy, which consists of standard occupational, physical, and speech therapies.

Discharged

Released from therapy. Discharged is the technical term that therapists use to describe the point at which therapy is ended. Different therapeutic disciplines (e.g., physical, occupational, speech therapy) may end at different times, depending on the progression, or lack of progression, of the stroke survivor. Therapists will usually continue therapy until they perceive that progress toward recovery has ended. Therapists call this lack of progress a **plateau**. The point at which any patient is discharged for any therapy is also dictated by the strict parameters set up by insurance companies, both private and governmental.

Distributed practice

A schedule of practice in which learning a new movement or skill is spread out over time. Distributed practice schedules are typically used in rehabilitation facilities. For instance, a typical rehabilitation schedule might be three sessions per week, 45 minutes each session, or five sessions a week for 1 hour. Contrast with **massed practice**.

Dorsiflexion

The movement of the foot upward when only the ankle joint is moved. If you are sitting in a chair with your feet on the ground and you want to tap your foot, the first movement of the foot, upward, is dorsiflexion. In many stroke survivors, this movement is limited or lost. The verb is "dorsiflex." A lack of ability to dorsiflex is called **drop foot** or **foot drop.**

Drop foot or foot drop

A reduced or eliminated ability to lift (dorsiflex) the foot at the ankle.

Dysarthria

Weakness or paralysis of the muscles of the mouth that form words. Dysarthria refers to impairments in speech caused by a reduced ability to use the muscles associated with speech. Dysarthria may affect the muscles of the mouth, lips, tongue, face, and respiratory system. Dysarthria is caused by damage, from the stroke, to the part of the brain that controls the movement of the mouth. Dysarthria can be reduced by the same mechanisms that reduce disability in the limbs, including **repetitive practice.** Contrast with **expressive aphasia.**

Electrical stimulation

See *neuromuscular electrical stimulation.*

Electrical stimulation ankle-foot orthosis (or "orthotics")

A group of commercially available orthotics designed to use electrical stimulation to lift the foot (**dorsiflexion**) in people with drop foot.

Embolitic stroke

A stroke caused by an embolism (usually a blood clot) that travels from another part of the body and lodges in and clogs an artery leading to the brain or in the brain. The embolism cuts off the blood supply to part of the brain, causing stroke.

Electromyography (EMG)

The testing of muscles as they contract (flex) and relax. Electromyography is often used to evaluate spastic muscles. It is also used in some electrical stimulation stroke-recovery machines to provide feedback to the machine regarding the amount of muscular effort by the stroke survivor.

Electromyography (EMG)-based electrical stimulation

Electrical stimulation that "rewards" the stroke survivor who tries to move a limb that is (or nearly is) immobile. If the stroke survivor tries to move the limb, electrical stimulation is sent to the muscles that complete the desired movement. Some of these machines are quite sensitive and can detect a signal even when no movement is visually apparent. Machines in this class include the Mentamove, The Biomove 3000 system, and NeuroMove™.

E-stim

Electrical stimulation. See *neuromuscular electrical stimulation.*

Evidence-based practice

Basing treatment of a patient on the best available research, as well as sound clinical judgment. It is of considerable benefit for stroke survivors to make sure that the treatment techniques they are using, with or without the administration by a therapist, are evidence based.

Expressive aphasia

The loss or limitation of communicating, either through the spoken word or the written one. Expressive aphasia is caused by damage to the language centers of the brain. Stroke survivors sometimes have expressive aphasia if they have had a left-sided stroke (right side of the body affected).

FES

See *functional electrical stimulation.*

Foot drop

An inability to **dorsiflex** (lift the foot at the ankle).

Functional

A term used by insurance companies and therapists to describe the ability to do a real-world task. For instance, if stroke survivors are able to dress themselves, no matter how they do it, they are said to be functional in dressing. The word "functional" does not necessarily address the deficits of the affected ("bad") side of the stroke survivor.

Functional electrical stimulation

Low levels of electrical stimulation run from a machine, through wires, and into electrodes put on the surface of the skin overlying the muscles involved in a functional task. The electricity contracts the muscles in a precise pattern that allows for a specific task to be accomplished.

Greater trochanter

A large bump that is at the top of the femur (the large bone that forms the top half of the leg). This bump is the surface that often hits the ground first when someone with a stroke falls. Discrete hip pads that can be worn inside undergarments will protect the vulnerable part of the hip during a fall.

Hemiparesis

Half the body is partially paralyzed. Hemiparesis is often incorrectly used to describe **hemiplegia.**

Hemiplegia

Total paralysis of the head, arm, leg, and trunk on one side of the body, whereas **hemiparesis** is weakness on one side of the body. Hemiplegia is often incorrectly used to describe hemiparesis.

Hemorrhagic stroke

A stroke in which a blood vessel bursts and blood is released into the brain. Hemorrhagic strokes make up approximately 20% of all strokes. The classic question to determine the type of stroke that a stroke survivor had is, "Was your stroke a bleed (hemorrhagic) or a block (**is-chemic**)?"

Home Exercise Program (HEP)

Traditionally, therapists have viewed the home exercise program (HEP) as a series of exercises that followed two rules: 1) The exercises given to the stroke survivor right before the therapist discharged the survivor; 2) the exercises were the same exercises that the stroke survivor had done with the therapist in the clinic. These are the same exercises that have precipitated the plateau that has caused the survivor to be discharged. If done correctly, a HEP can provide two important ingredients to the process of recovery: 1) A robust HEP can allow the survivor to continue to recover even after they've been discharged from therapy. 2) While in therapy with the therapists, a HEP can expand the amount of practice time per day. In this way the HEP expands the therapeutic experience the same way a child's homework expands the time allotted to learning a subject.

Imagery

See *mental practice.*

Ischemic stroke

A stroke in which blood is blocked from going through an artery that leads to or resides in the brain. The way the artery is blocked further distinguishes between two separate types of ischemic strokes: 1) **throm-botic stroke,** 2) **embolic stroke.**

Learned nonuse

The result of trying and failing a movement so often that the stroke survivor believes that the effort is futile. With lack of attempt comes shrinkage of the part of the brain that was used for that movement prior to the stroke. Researchers believe that survivors can overcome learned nonuse with interventions that force use, such as **constraint-induced therapy**.

Mass synergies

A large set of movements where no single movement can be done alone. In stroke survivors, during some periods in the arc of recovery, movements cannot be isolated. That is, stroke survivors cannot just do one movement (e.g., bend their elbow) without doing a whole series of movements (e.g., raising and bringing back the shoulder and the upper arm coming away from the body, etc.). All the movements, when taken together, defines mass synergies.

Massed practice

A schedule of practice in which learning a new movement or skill is done many hours a day, usually over a 2- to 3-week period. Massed-practice schedules are not typically used in rehabilitation facilities. However, **constraint-induced therapy** (CIT) is usually done using a massed-practice schedule. Constraint-induced therapy has traditionally used a schedule of 5 to 8 hours per day, for 2 to 3 weeks. Contrast with **distributed practice**.

Melodic intonation therapy (MIT)

A speech therapy that uses simple and exaggerated melodic elements to recreate speech. Because the area of the brain that typically processes music is on the opposite side of the brain that typically processes language, MIT aims to use nondamaged parts of the brain to compensate for the language areas of the brain affected by stroke.

Mental practice

A technique long used by athletes and musicians to precisely imagine physical movements in an attempt to enhance performance during the actual event. Traditionally known as "imagery," mental practice consists of deep relaxation followed by a disciplined practice of imagining moving the same way as prior to the stroke. Research indicates that mental practice may increase quality of movement in stroke survivors.

Meta-analysis

A meta-analysis is, essentially a "study of studies" where all the available studies of a subject are evaluated based on a set of pre-established criterion. Once the studies are evaluated, they are given a certain weight and run through a mathematical formula. A meta-analysis dedicated to stroke recovery gives scores to all the recovery strategies for which there is available research and distinguishes "winners" from "lemons." The definitive stroke-recovery meta-analysis is the Evidence-based Review of Stroke Rehabilitation by Dr. Robert Teasell and colleagues at the University of Western Ontario, Canada. This amazing stroke-specific document can be found on the web at www.ebrsr.com.

Mirror therapy

A therapy in which the stroke survivor copies the movement of the "good" upper extremity with the "bad" extremity while looking at the unaffected side through a mirror. The mirror gives the optical illusion that the affected extremity is moving perfectly. This therapy is thought to provide the brain with fake, but normalizing, information, fooling the brain into rewiring in a way that allows for more normal movement.

Modified constraint-induced therapy (mCIT)

A form of **constraint-induced therapy** that uses a schedule that is available within the normal schedule of typical outpatient settings. Developed by noted stroke researcher Dr. Stephen Page, mCIT involves the stroke survivor seeing a therapist three times a week for half-hour sessions. At home, the stroke survivor constrains the affected arm for 5 hours during a time when he or she is wakeful and active. Many rehabilitation facilities have modified mCIT even further, in order to reflect the particular skill of their therapists and to reflect the particular resources available at their facilities.

Necessity drives recovery

A phrase that describes the fact that *needing* to do a valued, real-world task (necessity) promotes recovery. The more essential a task is to a survivor, the more the task can be used to focus efforts toward accomplishment of the task.

Neuro

A prefix that means "nerve." Neuro is used as a prefix for anything that has to do with nerves, as in neurorecovery or **neuroplasticity**. Stroke is damage to the nerves of the brain.

Neuromuscular electrical stimulation (NMES)

The sort of electrical stimulation that causes muscles to contract. A machine delivers specific amounts of electrical stimulation down a wire and into an electrode that, with the use of a sticky gel, attaches to the skin overlying the muscles that are to be stimulated. Even muscles that are paralyzed after stroke respond to NMES. This treatment has shown promise as a way of retaining range of motion, muscle strength, and may even help jump start movement in **paretic** limbs. Neuromuscular electrical stimulation can be used in the arm or leg. Many companies are developing machines that provide NMES in orthotics, which allow the stroke survivor to move and practice everyday tasks, often with independence from tethering wires.

Neuroplasticity, neuroplastic, neuroplastically

The ability for neurons (nerve cells) to communicate with each other in new and ever-changing ways. Research using brain-imaging techniques has shown that neuroplasticity allows stroke survivors to recover by rearranging neuronal connections to "go around" the area of the brain damaged by stroke. It has been demonstrated that with the correct type, intensity, and schedule of practice, neuroplasticity can reallocate a part of the brain to any task practiced.

Paralysis

The complete loss of muscle control

Paresis, paretic

Partial loss of muscle control. The adjective is paretic.

Partial weight-supported walking (PWSW)

Walking while part of the weight of the stroke survivor is reduced, which lessens the effect of gravity and protects the stroke survivor if balance is lost. The reduction of body weight can be accomplished in two ways:

Having the stroke survivor wear a harness that is attached to risers. The risers are attached to a suspension device so that the stroke survivor can be suspended over a treadmill.

Having the stroke survivor supported through the pelvis in a mobile wheeled device. Once the stroke survivor is secure in the device, the device provides adequate lift to allow walking over ground. The KineAssist™ and NeuroGym® Bungee Walker are examples of this technology.

Partial weight-supported treadmill training

The stroke survivor wears a harness attached to risers that are then attached to a suspension device so that the stroke survivor can be suspended over a treadmill on which he or she walks.

Passive movement

Movement that is not performed by the person's own muscular power. For example, passive movement of the elbow would involve someone besides the stroke survivor moving the joint. However, passive movement can be done by the stroke survivor him- or herself, as well. For instance, if the stroke survivor moves the affected elbow with the unaffected hand, then the "bad" elbow is said to be involved in passive movement. Passive movement of the affected limbs is often an important part of reducing the risk of contracture and retaining **passive range of motion**. Some research indicates that passive movement may drive positive neuroplastic change.

Passive range of motion (PROM)

The amount of movement available in a joint when the joint is moved with **passive movement**. For example, the PROM of the elbow would be the amount of movement measured from the angle of the most flexion (elbow bent) to the angle of the elbow when it is most extended (elbow straight).

Patient driven

The term used to describe two separate ideas:
- **Neuroplasticity** in the brain is "driven" by the stroke survivor. Stroke survivors "drive" their own nervous systems during voluntary effort, and through this process, neuroplastic changes in the brain occur.
- Therapies are said to be "patient driven" when, with little training and/or set-up, the patient can do the therapies by themselves.

Peer-reviewed

The term used for research articles that have been scrutinized by experts in the field. For instance, an article about a new treatment for the recovery from stroke might be published in a peer-reviewed journal. If so, this article has a high chance of being accurate and reliable. However, much of what is published, either in books, newspapers, and magazines, and on the Internet does not go through the peer-review process and, therefore, is not considered as reliable as peer-reviewed information. If the source is simply reporting what a peer-reviewed article said, then it may be a reliable resource. Keep in mind that the mainstream media may misinterpret what was originally published in a peer-reviewed article. In any case, when researching different ways of recovering from stroke, look for information that was originally published in journals that are peer-reviewed.

Penumbra

The area next to the part of the brain killed by the stroke. The penumbra is often said to contain cells that are "stunned"—not dead, but not functioning. In the early stages after stroke, the penumbra begins to resolve, and as it does, recovery is often rapid.

Percutaneous

A medical procedure, where the skin is punctured to access tissue under the skin.

Percutaneous NMES (perc-NMES)

A form of **neuromuscular electrical stimulation** where the stimulation is delivered under the skin to the muscles. For instance, percutaneous electrical stimulation is sometimes used to reduce shoulder **subluxation** (shoulder dislocation) after stroke.

Physiatrist

A medical doctor specifically trained in physical medicine and rehabilitation. Often called "stroke doctors" by stroke survivors, these doctors have special medications, measurements, and treatments to help stroke survivors recover.

Plateau, plateaued

A word that means "flattening out," used to describe the point at which a stroke survivor is no longer making progress. Different therapeutic interventions (e.g., physical, occupational, and speech therapy) may plateau at different times. A plateau in progress may be more reflective of ineffective treatment options, ineffective implementations of treatment options, or incorrect dosages, rather than an actual halting of potential.

Proprioception

The feeling of where parts of the body (e.g., arms and legs) are in space without actually looking at the specific body part. The information about where the body is in space is delivered to the brain from little organs in the muscle and tendons called proprioceptors.

Range of motion (ROM)

The largest arc of movement of a joint. Range of motion is broken down into two categories; **active range of motion (AROM)** and **passive range of motion (PROM)**.

Reciprocal innervation

A phenomenon first described by Nobel laureate Sir Charles Sherrington that describes the fact that for a muscle (agonist) to contract, the muscle that opposes that muscle (antagonist) has to relax. For instance, in order for the muscles that bend the elbow to work, the muscles that straighten the elbow must "agree" to relax. This intricate dance between muscles is controlled subconsciously, by the spinal cord, not the brain.

Resistance training

Any training in which muscles work against an opposing force. The most common type of resistance training is weightlifting. This sort of exercise is essential to recovery from stroke.

Receptive aphasia

An inability to understand spoken language. Stroke survivors sometimes have receptive aphasia when they have had a left-sided stroke (right side of the body affected).

Repetitive practice

Repeating a movement or series of movements in order to drive neuroplastic change to benefit future attempts at the same movement.

Resolution of the penumbra

A reduction of swelling in the brain that leads to rapid recovery in the few weeks to months after the stroke. The **penumbra**, the area in which swelling is reduced, is next to the nerve cells in the brain killed by the stroke.

Rhythmic auditory cuing

Using a steady beat, generated by a metronome, drum machine, or music to establish a tempo that the stroke survivor tries to match by doing a particular movement or set of movements on the sound of the beat.

Rhythmicity, Rhythmic

The inherent rhythm in something. In recovery from stroke, rhythm can be used to motivate and provide an auditory cue. For instance, having one hand reach out and hit a target may help the stroke survivor learn to move. But if the same exercise is done while trying to hit the target on the snare beat for an entire song, then the exercise becomes motivating and more challenging.

Serial casting

A proven method for increasing the length of muscles shortened by spasticity and/or weakness. During serial casting, a cast is placed around a joint in a lengthened position so that the muscle is gradually and continually stretched.

Sherrington, Sir Charles

The scientist who, in the late 1800s and early 1900s, developed the foundation of modern physical and occupational therapy. In addition to a huge amount of neurological discoveries and observations, Nobel Prize winner Sherrington described **reciprocal innervation** and **proprioception,** two essential concepts in the recovery from stroke.

Soft tissue

The "meat" of the body that surrounds organs and bones. Included are muscles, tendons, ligaments, fat, fascia, nerve fibers, blood vessels, and joint tissue. In stroke survivors, soft tissue has the potential to irreversibly shorten because the affected joints are held in flexed postures. A comprehensive stretching program is essential to keeping soft tissue long enough so that, if and when control over the joints is reestablished, there is enough soft tissue length to accommodate the "new" movement. If soft tissue is not stretched enough, an irreversible shortening of soft tissue, called a **contracture**, can develop.

Spasticity, spastic

Tight and sometimes locked muscles caused by impulses from the spinal cord. The part of the brain that normally communicates with the muscles dies during the stroke. The muscles need protection from being torn, so the spinal cord sends endless signals to the muscles to contract. There are many temporary ways to reduce spasticity, including medications, but there is only one way to end spasticity: reestablishing brain control over the spastic muscles.

Speed-intensive gait training (SIGT)

Gait (walking) training that is done at speeds that are faster than typical gait training. Some researchers believe walking speed and quality will improve when gait training occurs at faster speeds.

Stretch reflex

The immediate muscle-protection reaction caused by impulses from the spinal cord. Stretch reflexes protect muscles from being over-stretched and torn. The patellar stretch reflex, in which a clinician will use a reflex hammer to tap just below the kneecap, is an example of a stretch reflex.

Stroke survivor

A person who has a stroke but does not die from the stroke.

Stages of recovery

See *Brunnstrom's stages of recovery.*

Subluxation of the shoulder

Dislocation of the shoulder joint as the head of the humerus (upper arm bone) separates from the glenoid fossa of the scapula (shoulder blade bone). Width of separation is usually measured in fingerbreadths. Shoulder subluxation may or may not be painful.

Synergistic movement

Movement that does not allow isolated movement of just one joint, but requires the movement of all the joints in the limb in order to perform that one movement. See also **Mass synergies** and **synergy**.

Synergy

The combination of more than one action that always happens together, usually in a complementary way. In stroke survivors, synergy is used to describe movements that are necessarily bundled together in a way that makes isolated moment impossible.

Task-oriented therapy

See *task-specific training.*

Task-specific training

The practicing of tasks that are meaningful to the stroke survivor. For instance, if a stroke survivor is a golfer, practice that involves some aspect of golf, or tasks that have the potential to lead to some aspect of the game of golf, are said to be task-specific. This sort of therapeutic intervention is known as task-specific training. In research with both humans and animals, it has been shown that therapy that incorporates tasks that are meaningful provide neuroplastic change along with increased active movement.

Thrombolytic stroke

A stroke caused by a clot formed inside a blood vessel in the brain or leading to the brain.

Treadmill training (TT)

A form of gait (walking) training that incorporates a treadmill. Treadmills offer "endless parallel bars," a predictable and nonslip walking surface, and gradation of incline or speed—all with indoor safety and comfort.

Tremor

Involuntary, usually rhythmic, movements.

Taub, Edward, PhD

The originator of **constraint-induced therapy**. Dr. Taub worked for decades with lab animals proving that constraint-induced therapy could work prior to introducing the therapy to human populations.

Waist-to-hip ratio

The relationship between the measurement of the stomach and the hips. To calculate, divide the measurement around the belly by the measurement around the hips. The belly is measured at the belly button, and the hips are measured around their widest point. The calculation is:

(Waist measurement) ÷ (Hip measurement) = (Waist-to-hip ratio)
There are many waist-to-hip ratio calculators on the web (Google: "waist-to-hip ratio calculator"). Research has shown that the waist-to-hip ratio is one of the best indicators of cardiac (heart attack) risk.

Wolf's Law

A widely accepted theory that the more stress put on a bone over time will reshape that bone to better handle that stress. Bone will get thicker and stronger if one does resistance exercises (weight training or working muscles against any resistance, e.g., gravity or resistance bands). Stroke survivors tend to have weaker bones (osteoporosis) on the affected side, coupled with the fact that when stroke survivors fall, they tend to fall toward the affected side. Since the bones on that side are weak, there is increased risk of fracture. Wolf's Law can be used to make bones thicker and stronger, reducing the risk of fracture.

INDEX

About the Author

Peter G. Levine is co-director of the Neuromotor Recovery and Rehabilitation Laboratory (rehablab.org) located in Drake Center, and under the auspices of the University of Cincinnati Academic Medical Center. He has been involved in stroke-specific rehabilitation research for more than a decade. Levine has co-authored articles in every major peer-reviewed journal that deals with neurological recovery in the United States and has authored articles in national magazines, including the National Stroke Association's magazine, *StrokeSmart* and writes a monthly column on stroke recovery in *Advance for Physical Therapists*. He conducts workshops throughout the United States for Education Resources Inc. (www.educationresourcesinc.com) in the area of stroke rehabilitation and neuroplasticity.

Before coming to the University of Cincinnati, Levine was a research associate in the Human Performance & Motion Analysis Laboratory at Kessler Rehabilitation Research and Education Corporation, the research division of the Kessler Institute for Rehabilitation.

Levine resides in Wyoming, Ohio, with his wife, Aila Mella (a physical therapist) and their two children. He can be reached via e-mail at **Stronger AfterStroke@yahoo.com.**

NOTES

NOTES

NOTES

NOTES

NOTES

Other Demos Titles for Stroke Survivors and Their Families

After a Stroke: 300 Tips for Making Life Easier, Cleo Hutton, 2005, 148 pages, ISBN 13: 978-1-932603-11-8

Stroke (American Academy of Neurology Series), Louis Caplan, MD, 2006, 256 pages, ISBN 13: 978-1-932603-14-9

101 Accessible Vacations: Travel Ideas for Wheelers and Slow Walkers, Candy B. Harrington, 2008, 352 pages, ISBN 13: 978-1-932603-43-9

There Is Room at the Inn: Inns and B&Bs for Wheelers and Slow Walkers, Candy B. Harrington, 2006, 256 pages, ISBN 13: 978-1-932603-61-3

Barrier-Free Travel: A Nuts and Bolts Guide for Wheelers and Slow Walkers, 2nd Edition, Candy B. Harrington, 2005, 304 pages, ISBN 13: 978-1-932603-09-5

The Personal Care Attendant Guide: The Art of Finding, Keeping, or Being One, Katie Rodriguez Banister, 2007, 170 pages, ISBN 13: 978-1-932603-28-6

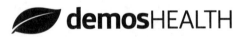 **demos**HEALTH

11W. 42nd Street, 15th Floor
New York, NY 10036
Tel: 800-532-8663 / 212-683-0072
Fax: 212-941-7842
www.demoshealth.com